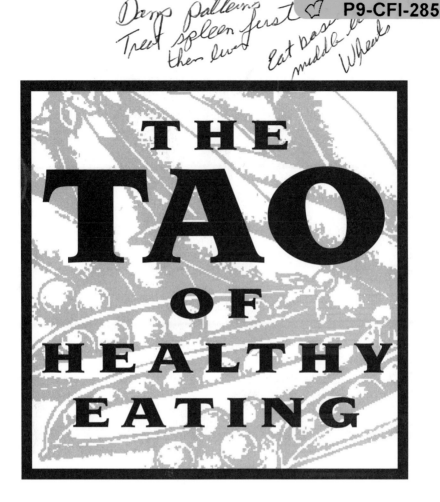

BOB FLAWS

BOULDER • COLORADO
BLUE POPPY PRESS

Other Books By
BOB FLAWS

Imperial Secrets of Health & Longevity

Keeping Your Child Healthy with Chinese Medicine

Curing Headaches Naturally with Chinese Medicine

Curing Fibromyalgia Naturally with Chinese Medicine

Curing Insomnia Naturally with Chinese Medicine

Curing Hay Fever Naturally with Chinese Medicine

Curing Arthritis Naturally with Chinese Medicine

THE TAO OF HEALTHY EATING

DIETARY WISDOM ACCORDING TO CHINESE MEDICINE

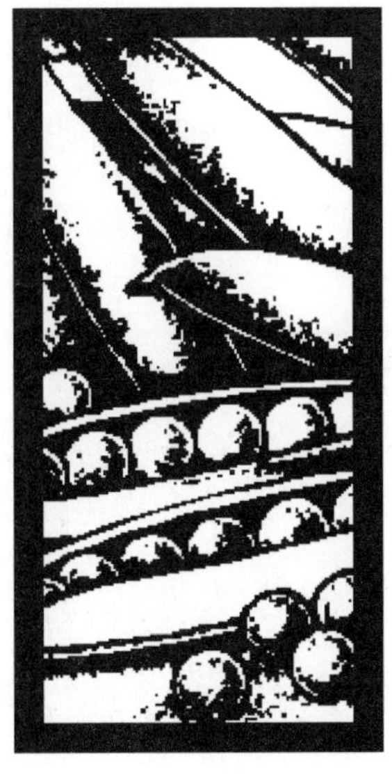

BOB FLAWS

Published by:
BLUE POPPY PRESS
A Division of Blue Poppy Enterprises, Inc.
3450 Penrose Place, Suite 110
Boulder, CO 80301

First Edition, January, 1998
Second Printing, August, 1998
Third Printing, August, 1999
Fourth Printing, July, 2001
Fifth Printing, July, 2002

ISBN 0-936185-92-9

WARNING: When following some of the self-care techniques given in this book, failure to follow the author's instruction may result in side effects or negative reactions. Therefore, please be sure to follow the author's instructions carefully for all self-care techniques and modalities. For instance, wrong or excessive application of moxibustion may cause local burns with redness, inflammation, blistering, or even possible scarring. If you have any questions about doing these techniques safely and without unwanted side effects, please see a local professional practitioner for instruction.

DISCLAIMER: The information in this book is given in good faith. However, the author and the publishers cannot be held responsible for any error or omission. The publishers will not accept liabilities for any injuries or damages caused to the reader that may result from the reader's acting upon or using the content contained in this book.

COMP Designation: Original work using a standard translational terminology

Printed at Johnson's Printing in Boulder, CO
on essentially chlorine-free paper
Book & cover design by Anne Rue
Cover illustration by Anne Rue

10 9 8 7 6 5

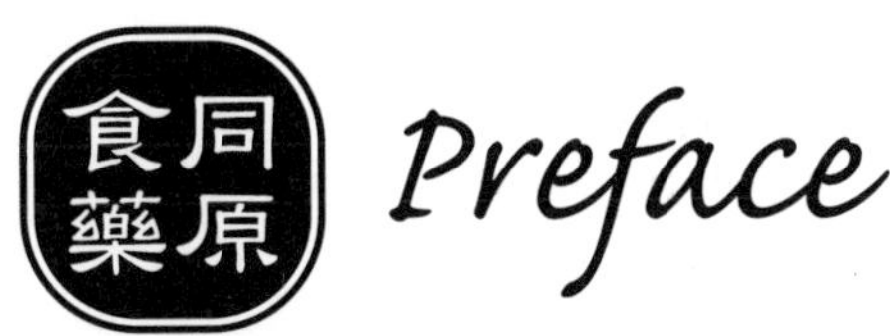

Preface

This small, concise book on Chinese dietary therapy has been written specifically for lay readers. It is meant to replace two earlier books I have written on Chinese dietary therapy, *Prince Wen Hui's Cook* and *Arisal of the Clear.* This book is a distillation of what I continually tell my patients day in and day out. I have tried to keep technical information to a minimum and have emphasized the use of simple metaphors to convey this information in an easily understandable way. Healthy eating is not all that complex or difficult to understand, and most people do not need extremely unique and unusual diets. The basic insights of traditional Chinese dietary therapy are relatively simple and universally applicable, especially within temperate regions.

Much of the information in this book was included in *Arisal of the Clear.* The main differences between that book and this are the inclusion of sections on the Chinese medical descriptions of nutritional supplements and the Chinese medical descriptions of over 150 foods commonly eaten in the West. These inclusions should make this book more useful to a wider group of readers.

I believe that Chinese dietary theory makes the most sense of any approach to healthy eating currently available. It explains digestion and nutrition in a very immediate, common sense, and human way. It also substantiates and helps make sense of many of the latest scientific opinions about food and diet. Hopefully, this book will fill the clear and present need for a concise layperson's guide to Chinese dietary therapy. If it does, then *bon appétit* and *wan sui*, good eating and may you live ten thousand years.

Bob Flaws
Boulder, CO
July 1997

食同
藥原

Table of Contents

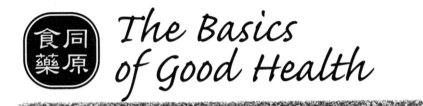

食同藥原 The Basics of Good Health

In the Tang Dynasty, the famous doctor Sun Si-miao said that, when a person is sick, the doctor should first regulate the patient's diet and lifestyle. In most cases, these changes alone are enough to effect a cure over time. Sun Si-miao said that only if changes in diet and lifestyle are not enough should the doctor administer other interventions, such as internal medicine and acupuncture. Although most patients coming for professional TCM treatment today do need internal medicine and/or acupuncture as well as changes in their diet and lifestyle to effect a more rapid cure, it is most definitely my experience that without appropriate changes in diet and lifestyle, herbs and acupuncture do not achieve their full and lasting effect.

Form & Function

There are four basic foundations of achieving and maintaining good health. These are diet, exercise, adequate rest and relaxation, and a good mental attitude. Chinese medical theory is based on yin and yang. In terms of medicine, yin means substance and yang means function. This is similar to the Western medical dichotomy between form and function. Form and function are interdependent. Substance or form is both the material, anatomical basis of function and its fuel. Function, on the other hand, activates and motivates form and also repairs, builds, and maintains it.

We can liken the human organism to a candle. A candle's function is to burn and, therefore, shed light. The flame of the candle is dependent upon its form. At the same time, the candle's form, its wick and wax, is the fuel for the candle's function. The human organism is very similar to a candle in that our various activities and consciousness are dependent upon our form, our physical body. Our functional activities are a product of consuming and transforming or metabolizing this substance. When we are young, we generate more substance than we consume and thus we are able to grow, repair, and keep our bodies youthful in shape and appearance. However, past a certain age, due to a decline in our bodily organs' efficiency, we no longer produce an excess of fuel or substance and so we begin to consume our own form. When we have consumed all our yin substance, our organism no longer has sufficient fuel for function and so ceases or dies.

Unlike the candle which is endowed with a finite, unreplenishable form at the moment of its making, we humans are capable of taking in new form or substance. We do this by breathing, eating, and drinking. It is eating and drinking which provide us with the substance which fuels our day to day activities and which is transformed into our body's material basis. Therefore, from the point of view of morphology or yin substance, we most definitely are what we eat, drink, and breathe.

Exercise is a form of function. It is activity. In relationship to diet, exercise is yang to diet's yin. Exercise keeps function functioning at peak efficiency. However, in Chinese medicine, exercise and rest/relaxation are seen as the yin/yang aspects of a single issue. If we are too active, *i.e.*, hyperfunctional, we consume too much fuel or substance. Therefore, rest and relaxation are the flip side of the coin of activity. Functional activities should be moderate—not too much and not too little. If there is too little exercise, form or material substance is not adequately consumed and transformed and starts to accumulate and gum up the works. If there is too little rest, hyperactivity, be that physical, mental, or emotional, consumes too much substance and overheats the organism leading to burnout. This means that diet on the one hand must be balanced by adequate activity and rest/relaxation on the other.

Fire & Essence

The use of a candle as an analogy is actually quite accurate according to Chinese medical theory. Life is seen in TCM as a series of warm transformations. The root yang of the entire body is called the *ming men zhi huo* or the fire of the gate of life. This life fire is responsible for all activities and transformations in the body. We live only as long as this fire of life burns within us and we are stone cold dead when it burns out irrevocably.

This life fire is associated with or has its material basis in the Chinese idea of the kidneys. In Chinese medicine, the kidneys are the fundamental, first organ. They are called the *xian tian zhi ben* or former heaven root. This means they are the prenatal foundation of the organism, both its form and function. The original source of function is the life fire described above. Whereas the most essential material basis or pure substance is referred to as the *jing* essence or *shen jing*, kidney essence.

In Chinese medicine, there are two types of *jing* essence. There is *xian tian zhi jing* or former heaven essence. This is innate at birth. We are born with a finite amount of this former heaven essence. It is our endowment from our parents and the universe at large and it is stored in the kidneys. This former heaven essence is supplemented by what is called *hou tian zhi jing* or latter heaven essence. This latter heaven essence is manufactured out of the air we breathe and the food and drink we consume. Nutritive essence derived from food is transformed into qi (pronounced chee) and blood. Qi empowers function and blood nourishes form. As we move through each day, our activities consume both qi and blood. If, when we go to sleep at night, we have manufactured more qi and blood than we have used that day, this excess is transformed into acquired or latter heaven essence. Some of this latter heaven essence is stored in each of the five major organs in Chinese medicine—the heart, lungs, spleen, liver, and kidneys. However the major portion of this acquired essence is stored in the kidneys which then form the Fort Knox of the body.

Every metabolic activity, every transformation within the organism requires both some life fire and some *jing* essence to act as catalyst and substrate respectively. If there were no acquired essence, we would be just like a candle. We would only be born with so much fuel and that would be used up fairly quickly. However, because latter heaven essence, derived from our diet, supplements our innate former heaven essence stored in our kidneys, this former heaven essence is capable of lasting a lifetime.

Longevity, Diet & Lifestyle

Chinese medical theory believes that the human organism is built to live 100 years. According to the first chapter of the *Nei Jing*, the premier classic of Chinese medicine, most people have enough *jing* essence to last 5 score years. Barring accidental death or infectious disease, we are designed to last 100 years as long as former heaven essence is not squandered by excessive consumption and as long as latter heaven or acquired essence is manufactured and stored to bolster and slow the use of former heaven essence. Since latter heaven essence is manufactured from the food and drink we ingest, it is no wonder that Chinese medical theory places such great importance on proper diet and promoting good digestion. Likewise, since acquired essence is stored in the kidneys at night when we sleep, it is no wonder why proper rest and sleep are important as well.

Former heaven essence is like a patrimony or trust fund we inherit at birth. Latter heaven essence is like money which we save in the bank. It is that part of our daily economy above and beyond our operating expenses. When we store it as acquired *jing* essence, it and our former heaven essence together become our body's capital. It is said in alchemy that it takes gold to make gold and that the more gold one has, the more one can make. When applied to our inner alchemy, our original gold is our *jing* essence, both former and latter heaven. When these two essences are full and abundant, organ function is strong, metabolism is efficient, and we generate a profit each day. Therefore, it takes *jing* to make *jing* and the more *jing* we have, the more we can make. When we age, however, instead of living on our interest, we run a negative daily balance and are forced to dip into our capital. Eventually we consume all our capital and we go bankrupt or die.

Essence, Qi, Spirit

It is said in Chinese that essence (material basis) becomes qi (functional activity) and when qi accumulates it becomes spirit. Spirit means consciousness and mental/emotional activities. Excessive thinking or excessive emotionality consume great stores of qi and, therefore, essence. That is why the fourth basic foundation of good health is a healthy mental attitude. What is meant by a good attitude in Chinese medicine is spelled out fairly exactly. When the seven emotions—joy, anger, grief, worry, fear, fright, and melancholy—are appropriate to their stimuli, these are natural subjective experiences and their experience is the purpose of life. Nonetheless, their experience does consume essence. Essence without spirit or mental activity is meaningless in human terms just as a candle which doesn't shed light is also useless. The consumption of essence through our conscious experience is what is called in Chinese our *shen ming. Shen* means spirit or consciousness. *Ming* means brilliance or light. Essence's purpose is to be transformed into the light of consciousness.

It is further said in Chinese that spirit should apprehend emptiness and that this apprehension should also be reduced to nothingness. This gets a little abstruse but is worth everyone's understanding, patient and practitioner alike. The apprehension of emptiness means that, through one's life experiences, one understands that nothing, whether internally experienced or externally existent, is permanent or real. If one feels any experience all the way to its depth, it becomes empty. All experiences are reducible to an essential emptiness. Not only are they fleeting but they are of a single, unexpressable, indescribable taste. No matter whether one experiences joy or anger, fear or sadness, these mental/emotional experiences are evanescent and in no way alter or affect the innate nature of the spirit.

When one understands that the spirit is inviolable, essentially unharmable, and indestructible, one's experience, whether of good or bad, becomes like a movie projected on a screen. The movie is not the screen and no matter what drama is enacted on the screen, the screen is not harmed or affected. If one can apprehend this, then, in Chinese, one can say that spirit apprehends the essential emptiness of experience. However, if one then becomes attached to this concept of emptiness, that itself can cause an obstruction to the free flow of reality. Therefore, it is further said that emptiness must also be understood as nothingness or no-thing-ness. When one does, this is the absolute good mental attitude which is ultimately healthy.

Deepak Chopra, in *Quantum Healing*, has discussed the therapeutic importance of apprehending this state of absolute emptiness which is uncolored by one's passing and ever-changing emotions, thoughts, and sensations. Ironically, this apprehension is in part dependent upon the consumption of essence. It is a fundamental axiom that essence is consumed by the aging process and that the signs and symptoms of aging are the signs and symptoms of the kidneys becoming empty and then becoming insufficient. However, this process results in experiences, and if one has enough experiences and also has enough consciousness to reflect deeply on those experiences, one will understand that, no matter how many times one has been happy or sad, in pleasure or in pain, essentially it has not indelibly colored nor permanently altered one's essential being. This is the wisdom that hopefully comes with old age. It is the wisdom of spontaneous nonattachment, equipoise, naturalness, and the willingness to let things be.

We all get old and we all die. We all experience pain as well as pleasure. These are inevitable. When we fail to recognize the naturalness of this condition and rather take it as a personal affront or attack, we run after pleasure and its means in order to avoid suffering at all cost. Paradoxically, this ceaseless running towards pleasure and running away from pain consumes essence and causes the very disease, suffering, and death we seek to avoid. It is transcendence of this rat-race which the wisdom of the East posits as a good, healthy mental attitude.

Because of the above interrelationships between essence, *qi*, and spirit, it is easy to see why diet, exercise, rest, and the development of such a good, healthy attitude are so important to achieving and maintaining good health. This book focuses on dietary therapy. That does not mean that diet is more important than the other three. The diseases of this time are often due to a lack of wisdom in all four of these crucial areas. Although the contemporary Western diet shows some signs of improving in recent years, it is not based on the most enlightened concepts. In addition, we tend to be too sedentary at the same time as being too mentally and emotionally stressed. And few of us can be said to have gained a mature mental equipoise.

It is relatively simple to say that one should get enough exercise and rest. And although Buddhists, Daoists, and Confucianists have filled libraries on how to achieve a good mental attitude, this is not something that can be well conveyed in a book. Diet, on the other hand, although seemingly open to a great deal of contradiction and confusion, is something which can be written about simply and clearly.

食同
藥原

The Process of Digestion

In Chinese, the digestive system is called the *xiao hua xi tong.* The words *xi tong* simply mean system but the words *xiao* and *hua* are more pregnant with meaning. *Xiao* means to disperse and *hua* means to transform. In Chinese medicine, digestion equals the dispersion of pure substances to be retained and impure substances to be excreted after these have undergone transformation. Therefore, the digestive tract is called the *xiao hua dao* or pathway of dispersion and transformation. In TCM we mostly describe the process of digestion in terms of the functions of the Chinese stomach and spleen. Once one understands the functions of the stomach-spleen according to TCM theory, Chinese dietary theory becomes very clear and logical.

Three Burners

The stomach and spleen are a yin yang pair. The stomach is one of the six hollow bowels and is relatively yang. The spleen is one of the five solid organs and is relatively yin. The stomach's function is to receive food and liquids and to "rotten and ripen" these. In Chinese medicine, the stomach is likened to a pot on a fire. As mentioned in the previous chapter, all physiological transformations in Chinese medicine are warm transformations. The body is seen as three alchemical retorts. These are called *jiao* or burners. There is an upper burner containing the heart and lungs, a middle burner containing the stomach and spleen, and a lower burner containing the kidneys, intestines, liver, and reproductive organs.

The Stomach as a Pot

The stomach is the pot of the middle burner and the spleen is both the fire under this pot and the distillation mechanism to which this pot is attached. Just as a mash rottens and ripens in a pot, so foods and liquids rotten and ripen within the stomach. In Chinese medical terms, this means that, as foods and liquids rotten and ripen, the pure and impure parts of these foods and liquids are separated or come apart. It is then the spleen's function to distill or drive off upwards the purest parts of foods and liquids, sending the pure part of foods up to the lungs and the pure part of liquids up to the heart. The pure part of foods or the five flavors become the basis for the creation of qi or vital energy within the lungs. The pure part of liquids becomes the basis for the creation of blood within the heart. The sending up of the pure part of the foods and liquids by the spleen is called ascension of the clear.

The stomach then sends down the impure parts of foods to be further transformed by the large intestine and the impure parts of liquids to be further transformed by the small intestine. In Chinese medicine, the large intestine's function is to reabsorb the pure part of the impure foods or solids. This becomes the postnatal or latter heaven fuel for kidney yang or the life fire. The small intestine's function is to reabsorb the pure part of the impure parts of liquids. This is transformed into the body's thick liquids, such as cerebrospinal and intra-articular fluids, and nourishes postnatal kidney yin. The large intestine conducts the impure of the impure solids down and out of the body as feces. The small intestine conducts the impure of the impure liquids to the bladder from whence they are excreted as urine. This sending down of the impure part of foods and liquids initiated by the stomach is called the descension of the turbid.

Therefore, in Chinese medicine, digestion is spoken of as the separation of the clear *(qing)* and turbid *(zhuo)*. This separation is dependent upon the *qi hua* or energy transformation of the middle burner or stomach/spleen and upon the spleen qi's ability to transport or *yun* foods and fluids. Hence, Chinese spleen function is summed up in the two words *yun* (transportation) and *hua* (transformation). *Yun hua* is the older, more traditional form of the modern term *xiao hua*.

The analogy of the cooking pot is very important. It is said in Chinese that the stomach fears or has an aversion to dryness. In other words, stomach function is dependent upon the creating of a mash or soup in its cauldron or pot. It is also said in Chinese that the spleen fears dampness. Since spleen function is likened to a fire under a pot distilling the essence from the mash held in the stomach, it is easy to understand that too much water or dampness can douse or injure that fire.

Using this analogy, it is simple and crucial to understand that the digestive process, according to Chinese medicine, consists of first creating a 100°F soup in the stomach, remembering that body temperature is 98.6°F. Whatever facilitates the creation of such a 100° soup in the stomach benefits digestion and whatever impedes or impairs the creation of a 100° soup in the stomach impedes or impairs digestion. This is basically true even from a Western medical perspective. Most of the insights and principles of Chinese dietary theory and therapy are logical extensions of this commonsense and irrefutable truth.

The Implications of this Process

Cooked vs. Raw Foods

First of all, TCM suggests that most people, most of the time, should eat mostly cooked food. Cooking is predigestion on the outside of the body to make food more easily digestible on the inside. By cooking foods in a pot on the outside of the body, one can initiate and facilitate the stomach's rottening and ripening in its pot on the inside of the body. Cold and raw foods require that much more energy to transform them into warm soup within the pot of the stomach. Since it takes energy or qi to create this warmth and transformation, the net profit from this transformation is less. Whereas, if one eats cooked foods at room temperature at least or warm at best, less spleen qi is spent in the process of digestion. This means that the net profit of digestion, *i.e.,* qi or energy, is greater.

The idea that eating cooked food is more nutritious than raw food flies in the face of much modern Western nutritional belief. Because enzymes and vitamins are destroyed by cooking, many people think it is healthier to eat mostly raw, uncooked foods. This seemingly makes sense only as long as one confuses gross income with net profit. When laboratory scientists measure the relative amounts of cooked and raw foods, they are not taking into account these nutrients' post-digestive absorption.

Let's say that a raw carrot has 100 units of a certain vitamin or nutrient and that a cooked carrot of the same size has only 80 units of that same nutrient. At first glance, it appears that eating the raw carrot is healthier since one would, theoretically, get more of that nutrient that way. However, no one absorbs 100% of any available nutrient in a given food. Because the vitamins and enzymes of a carrot are largely locked into hard to digest cellulose packets, when one eats this raw carrot, they may actually only absorb 50% of the available nutrient. The rest is excreted in the feces. But when one eats the cooked carrot, because the cooking has already begun the breakdown of the cellulose walls, one may absorb 65% of the available nutrient. In this case, even though the cooked carrot had less of this nutrient to begin with, net absorption is greater. The body's economy runs on net, not gross. It is as simple as that. Of course, we are talking about light cooking, and not reducing everything to an overcooked, lifeless mush.

This is why soups and stews are so nourishing. These are the foods we feed infants and those who are recuperating from illness. The more a food is like 100° soup, the easier it is for the body to digest and absorb its nutrients. The stomach-spleen expend less qi and, therefore, the net gain in qi is greater. This is also why chewing food thoroughly before swallowing is so important. The more one chews, the more the food is macerated and mixed with liquids, in other words, the more it begins to look like soup or stew.

Cold Food & Liquids

As a corollary of this, if we drink or eat chilled, cold, or frozen foods or drink iced liquids with our meals, we are only impeding the warm transformation of digestion. Cold obviously negates heat. And water puts out fire. This does not mean that such food and liquids are never digested, but it does mean that often they are not digested well. In Chinese medicine, if the stomach-spleen fail to adequately transport and transform foods and liquids, a sludge tends to accumulate just as it might in an incompletely combusting automobile engine. This sludge is called stagnant food and dampness in Chinese medicine.

Dampness & Phlegm

If the solid portions of food are jam-packed into the stomach or their digestion is impaired by cold and chilled foods and liquids or if too many hard to digest foods are eaten, stagnant food may accumulate in the stomach. The stomach tries all the harder to burn these off and becomes like a car stuck in overdrive. It becomes hotter in an attempt to burn off the accumulation. This often results in the stomach becoming chronically overheated. This, in turn, causes the stomach to register hunger which, in Chinese medicine, is a sensation of the stomach's heat. This hunger then results in eating more and more and a vicious loop is created. Overeating begets stagnant food which begets stomach heat which reinforces overeating. Further, persistent stomach heat may eventually waste stomach yin or fluids causing a chronic thirst and preference for cold drinks and chilled foods.

If the liquid portions of food and drink jam the transporting and transforming functions of the spleen, what is called the *qi ji* or qi mechanism in Chinese, these may accumulate as dampness. This plethora of water inhibits the spleen qi's warm transforming function in the same way that water inhibits or douses fire. Over time, this accumulated dampness may mix with stagnant food and congeal into phlegm which further gums up the entire system and retards the flow of qi and blood throughout the body.

Different people's digestion burns hotter than others'. Those with a robust constitution and strong *ming men* or fire of life tend to have a strong digestion. These people can often eat more in general and more chilled, frozen, hard to digest foods without seeming problems. Likewise, everyone's metabolism runs at different temperatures throughout the year. During the summer when it is hot outside, we generally can eat cooler foods and should drink more liquids.

However, even then, we should remember that everything that goes down our gullet must be turned into 100° soup before it can be digested and assimilated.

Post-digestive Temperature

In Chinese medicine, there is an important distinction made between the cold physical temperature of a food or drink and a food or drink's post-digestive temperature. Post-digestive temperature refers to a particular food or drink's net effect on the body's thermostat. Some foods, even when cooked, are physiologically cool and tend to lower the body's temperature either systemically or in a certain organ or part. In Chinese medicine, every food is categorized as either cold, cool, level (*i.e.*, balanced or neutral), warm, or hot. Most foods are cool, level, or warm and, in general, we should mostly eat level and warm foods since our body itself is warm. Life is warm. During the winter or in colder climates, it is important to eat warmer foods, but during the summer we can and should eat cooler foods. However, this mostly refers to the post-digestive temperature of a food.

If one eats ice cream in the summer, the body at first is cooled by the ingestion of such a frozen food. However, its response is to increase the heat of digestion in order to deal with this cold insult. Inversely, it is a common custom in tropical countries to eat hot foods since the body is provoked then to sweat as an attempt to cool itself down. In China, mung bean soup and tofu are eaten in the summer because both these foods tend to cool a person down post-digestively. If we are going to eat cold and frozen foods and drink iced, chilled liquids, it is best that these be taken between meals when they will not impede and retard the digestion of other foods.

Many Westerners are shocked to think that cold and frozen foods are inherently unhealthy since they have become such an ubiquitous part of our contemporary diet. However, chilled, cold, and frozen foods and liquids are a relatively recent phenomenon. They are dependent upon refrigeration in the marketplace, refrigeration during transportation, and refrigeration in the home. Such mass access to refrigeration is largely a post World War II occurrence. That means that, in temperate zones, people have only had widespread access to such foods and drinks for less than 50 years. Fifty years is not even a blink on the human evolutionary scale.

Dampening Foods

Not only do foods have an inherent post-digestive temperature but different foods also tend to generate more or less body fluids. Therefore, in Chinese medicine, all foods can be described according to how damp they are, meaning dampening to the human system. Because the human body is damp, most foods are somewhat damp. We need a certain amount of dampness to stay alive. Dampness in food is yin in that dampness nourishes substance which is mostly wet and gushy. However, some foods are excessively dampening, and, since it is the spleen which is averse to dampness, excessively damp foods tend to interfere with digestion.

According to Chinese five phase theory, dampness is associated with earth. Fertile earth is damp. The flavor of earth according to Chinese five phase correspondence theory is sweet. The sweet flavor is inherently damp and also is nutritive. In Chinese medical terms, the sweet flavor supplements the qi and blood. Qi is energy or vital force and blood in this case stands for all body fluids. Therefore, the sweeter a food or liquid is, the more damp it tends to be.

When one looks at a Chinese medical description of various foods, one is struck by the fact that almost all foods are somewhat sweet and also supplement qi and blood. On reflection, this is obvious. We eat to replenish our qi and blood. Therefore it is no wonder most foods are somewhat sweet. All grains, most vegetables, and most meats eaten by humans are sweet no matter what other of the five flavors they may also be. This sweetness in the overwhelming majority of foods humans regularly eat becomes evident the more one chews a food.

A modicum of sweetness supplements the body's qi and blood. It is this flavor which gathers in the spleen and provides the spleen with its qi. However, excessive sweetness has just the opposite effect on the spleen. Instead of energizing the spleen, it overwhelms and weakens it. This is based on the Chinese idea that yang when extreme transforms into yin and vice versa. When the spleen becomes weak, it craves sweetness since that is the flavor which strengthens it when consumed in moderate amounts. However, if this craving is indulged with concentrated sweets, such as sugar, this only further weakens the spleen and harms digestion. Thus, another pathological loop is forged in many people.

Going back to dampness, the sweet flavor engenders dampness and the sweeter a food is the more dampening it is. According to Chinese medicine, this tendency is worsened when the sweet flavor is combined with sour. Therefore, Chinese medicine identifies a number of especially dampening foods. These include such sweet and sour foods as citrus fruits and juices and tomatoes, such concentrated sweets as sugar, molasses, and honey, and such highly nutritious foods as wheat, dairy products, nuts, oils, and fats.

Highly nutritious foods are those which have more *wei* than qi. All foods are a combination of qi and *wei.* In this context, qi means the light, airy, aromatic and yang part of a food. Whereas, *wei,* literally meaning taste, refers to a food's heavier, more substantial, more nourishing, yin aspects. Highly nutritious foods, such as dairy products, meats, nuts, eggs, oils, and fats are strongly capable of supplementing the body's yin fluids and substances. However, in excess, they generate a superabundance of body fluids which become pathologic dampness. Although to some this may appear a paradox, it has to do with healthy yin in excess becoming evil or pathological yin or dampness, phlegm, and turbidity.

It is also easy to see that certain combinations are even worse than their individual constituents. Ice cream is a dietary disaster. It is too sweet, too creamy, and too cold. Ice cream is a very, very dampening food. Pizza is a combination of tomato sauce, cheese, and wheat. All of these foods tend to be dampening and this effect is made even worse if greasy additions, such as pepperoni and sausage, are added. Tomato sauce bears a few more words. It is the condensed nutritive substances of a number of tomatoes. Therefore it can be especially dampening.

In the same way, drinking fruit juices can be very dampening. Fruit and vegetable juices are another relatively modern addition to the human diet. Prior to the advent of refrigeration as discussed above, juices would turn into wine or vinegar within days. Therefore, when they were available in traditional societies, they were an infrequent treat. Now we have access to tropical fruits and juices thanks to refrigeration and interstate and intercontinental transportation. However, we should bear in mind that we would not eat 4-6 oranges in a single sitting nor every day. When we drink a glass of orange juice, tomato juice, apple juice, or carrot juice, that is exactly what we are doing. We are drinking the nutritive essence of not one but a number of fruits or vegetables. This over-nutrition typically results in the formation of pathogenic dampness and phlegm.

Meats, because they are so nutritious, or supplement qi and blood so much, also tend to be damp in the same way. The fatter and richer a meat is, the more it tends to generate dampness within the body. Amongst the common domestic mammalian meats, pork is the dampest with beef coming in second. Therefore, it is important not to eat too much meat and especially not greasy, fatty meats. Most people do fine on two ounces of meat 3-4 times per week.

On the other hand, eating only poultry and fish is not such a good idea either. Everything in this world has its good and bad points. Poultry and fish tend to be less dampening and phlegmatic, it is true, but chicken, turkey, and shellfish tend to be hot. If one eats only these meats, they run the risk of becoming overheated. I have seen this happen in clinical practice. From a Western scientific point of view, we can also say that eating too much fish may result in mercury accumulation and toxicity and overeating commercial chicken may result in too much estrogen and exposure to salmonella food-poisoning. Chinese medicine sees human beings as omnivores and suggests that a person should eat widely and diversely on the food chain.

The Basic Healthy Diet

Therefore, to sum up the traditional wisdom of Chinese dietary theory, humans should mostly eat vegetables and grains with small amounts of everything else. We should mostly eat cooked and warm food which is not too sweet, not too greasy or oily, and not too damp. In addition, we should eat moderately and chew well. It is healthful to drink a teacup of warm water or a warm beverage with meals. This facilitates the formation of that 100° soup. But it is unhealthy to drink or eat chilled, cold, and frozen drinks and foods with meals.

In general, I would emphasize that most Americans do not eat enough vegetables. It is easy to load up on breads, grains, and cereals but not as easy to eat plenty of freshly cooked vegetables. Grains, like meat and dairy products, are highly nutritious but heavy and relatively more difficult to digest. If overeaten they can cause accumulation of dampness and phlegm. In Asia, Daoists and Buddhists interested in longevity emphasized vegetables over grains and even modern Chinese books on geriatrics counsel that more vegetables should be eaten.

Amongst the grains, rice holds an especially healthy place. Because it promotes diuresis, it tends to leech off excessive dampness. Other grains, in comparison, tend to produce dampness as a by-product of their being so nutritious. This ability of rice to help eliminate dampness through diuresis becomes more important the more dampening foods one eats.

Flavors & Spices

As said at the beginning of this chapter, the purest part of foods are the five flavors. These are sweet, salty, bitter, pungent, and sour. Chinese medicine also recognizes a sixth flavor called bland. Each of the five flavors corresponds to one of the five phases and, therefore, tends to accumulate and have an inordinate effect on one of the five major organs of Chinese medicine. Just as overeating sweet injures the spleen, overeating salt injures the kidneys, overeating sour injures the liver, and overeating spicy foods injures the lungs. I know of no one who overeats bitter food. A little bitter flavor is good for the heart and stomach. In general, although most food is sweet, one should eat a modicum of all the other flavors. Overeating any one flavor will tend to cause an imbalance in the organs and tissues associated with that flavor according to five phase correspondence.

Most spices are pungent or acrid and warm to hot. These spices aid digestion when eaten in moderate amounts. As discussed above, the digestive process is like an alchemical distillation. The middle burner fire of the stomach-spleen cooks and distills foods and liquids driving off their purest parts. To have good digestion means to have a healthy digestive fire. Moderate use of acrid, warm spices aids digestion by strengthening the middle burner fire.

That is why traditional cultures found the use of pepper, cardamom, cinnamon, ginger, nutmeg, mace, and cloves so salutary. These spices contain a high proportion of qi to *wei* and so help yang qi transform and distill yin substance, dampness, and fluids. On the other hand, when eaten to excess, such spices can cause overheating of the stomach and drying out of stomach fluids, and remember, the stomach does not like to be dry. Therefore, a moderate use of such spices is good for the spleen but their overuse is bad for the stomach and lungs.

A Return to a More Traditional Diet

What this all adds up to is a diet very similar to the Pritikin diet or Macrobiotics. Both these dietary regimes suggest that the bulk of one's diet be composed of complex carbohydrates and vegetables and that one get plenty of fiber and less animal proteins, refined sugars, oils, and fats. This is very much the traditional diet of all people living in temperate climates the world round. This is also very much like what our great grandparents ate.

One hundred years ago, most people only ate meat once or twice a week. Mostly they ate grains and vegetables. Because they did not have refrigeration, they ate mostly what was in season and what could be stored in root cellars and through pickling, salting, and drying. One hundred years ago, sugar was too expensive for most people to afford more than a tiny bit per year. Likewise, oils and fats were relatively precious commodities and were not eaten in large quantities. Those oils which were available were pressed from flax, hemp, sesame seeds, or were derived from fish oil, lard, and butter. They were not the heavily hydrogenated tropical oils which are so frequently used in commercial food preparation today.

It was also a well-known fact of life 100 years ago that rich people who ate too well and exercised too little were more prone to chronic health problems than those who lived a more spartan and rigorous life. If one looks at the cartoons of the 18th and 19th centuries, one frequently sees the overweight nobleman with the enlarged and gouty toe. Likewise, the Chinese medical classics contain numerous stories of doctors treating rich patients by getting them to do some physical work and to eat simpler, less rich food. Gerontologists today have noted the fact that those ethnic groups who tend to produce a large proportion of centenarians, such as the Georgians, the Hunzakuts, and certain peoples in the Peruvian Andes, all eat a low animal protein, low fat, high fiber diet.

The Modern Western Diet

The modern Western diet which we take so much for granted is mostly a product of post World War II advances in technology and transportation. Until after World War II, the lack of mass refrigeration and interstate transportation did not allow for everyone to buy a half gallon of fresh orange juice anytime of the year at an affordable price nor to keep a half gallon of ice cream (or now frozen yogurt) in their home freezer. In addition, special interest advertising has fostered erroneous ideas about the healthfulness of many of these "new" foods. We have been so bombarded by TV commercials extolling the healthful benefits of orange juice that we seldom remember that these are partisan propaganda bought and paid for by commercial growers who depend upon the sale of their product to turn a profit.

The modern Western diet is a relatively recent aberration in the history of human diet. It is an experiment which has largely run its course as more and more people as well as governmental agencies come to the conclusion that so much of what we take for granted these days as a normal diet is really not healthy. Just as we are now realizing as a society that smoking is bad for the health, likewise we are also now coming to realize that too much sugar, fats, oils, and animal protein are also not good for the health nor conducive to longevity.

Pesticides, Preservatives, & Chemicals

Traditional Chinese Medicine has, in the past, not said anything about pesticides, preservatives, and chemical additives because these things were not known until relatively recently. However, poisoning is a TCM cause of disease listed in the *bu nei bu wai yin* category of neither internal nor external etiologies. All the evidence suggests that eating food which is contaminated by pesticides, preservatives, and chemical dyes and additives is also not good for long term health and well being. Therefore, it is advisable to eat food which is as free from these as possible. That means organic produce and grains and organically grown meat. These are becoming increasingly more common and available.

Wrecked Foods

Since Chinese medicine says that the qi comes from the purest of the pure part of foods, the *xiang* or flavor/aroma, Chinese dietary theory also suggests that food should be freshly made and eaten within 24 hours. As food becomes stale, it loses its aroma and its ability to supplement qi is directly proportional to this aroma. Food which is stale is called wrecked food in Chinese. The implication is that, although the substance is still there, the *xiang*, aroma, or qi is gone. Such wrecked foods tend to be more dampening and phlegmatic.

If one follows the above Chinese dietary guidelines, one will eat nutritiously and well. One will be supplemented by their food and not unduly harmed by it. Such a moderate, commonsense diet is one of the four foundations of good health. This diet is more or less appropriate to everyone living in a temperate climate. Patients suffering from specific diseases may require various individualized modifications of the above outlined regime. However, because whether in sickness or health the process of digestion is essentially the same, this is the healthy diet for the majority of people. In the following chapter, we will discuss specific modifications for the most common groups of imbalance described by TCM. Yet even these modifications are based on this same commonsense approach to food and eating.

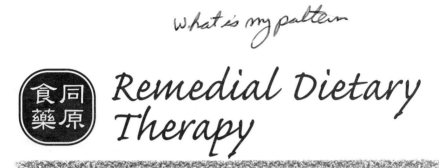

Remedial Dietary Therapy

There are three main principles to Chinese dietary therapy when it comes to the remedial treatment of disease which has already arisen.

1. Treatment should primarily be based on pattern discrimination

The first of these principles is to select foods which correspond to the patient's pattern. The hallmark of TCM as a style of medicine is that it primarily bases its treatment on the person's pattern rather than on their disease. A disease is usually defined by a small group of signs and symptoms. For instance, you cannot be diagnosed as having a headache if you do not have any pain in your head. However, different people may all be diagnosed as suffering from headache, but those different people may each suffer from a different type and severity of pain in different locations of their head. Further, they may be fat or thin, male or female, old or young, and have any number of other, unique, individualized complaints. A TCM pattern is the entire constellation of all a person's signs and symptoms and not just those that add up to their disease diagnosis.

Thus, it is said in Chinese medicine:

> *One disease, different treatments,*
> *Different diseases, one treatment.*

This means that if two patients both suffer from the same disease but exhibit different patterns of overall signs and symptoms, they will receive different TCM treatments; while two patients with different disease diagnoses may receive the same treatment if their TCM pattern is the same.

Therefore, we can say that treatment in TCM is aimed at remedying patterns and not diseases. In Chinese medicine, disease is seen as an imbalance. This imbalance may be between the various types of qi in the body, between the viscera and bowels, or between the various types of body fluids. The name of every TCM pattern is a description of how that person is out of balance. If a person is described as exhibiting a spleen qi vacuity weakness, this means that their spleen is not functioning up to par. The treatment principles necessary to correct that imbalance and restore the person to health are to fortify the spleen and supplement or boost the qi. In this case, the Chinese doctor knows that anything which accomplishes these two goals will be good for the patient, but anything which damages the spleen or weakens the qi further will make them worse.

In terms of remedial Chinese dietary therapy, this means that foods are selected on the basis of whether they help or hinder the restoration of the patient's overall pattern to a state of balance or health. Those which promote a movement back to balance should be eaten and those which aggravate the person's imbalance should be avoided. Thus the *Nei Jing*, the premier classic of Chinese medicine says, "If there is heat, cool it; if there is cold, warm it; if there is dryness, moisten it; if there is dampness, dry it; if there is vacuity, supplement it; and if there is repletion [*i.e.*, excess or fullness], drain it." Based on this saying, if one has a hot pattern, one should eat cool or cold, heat-clearing foods. But if one has a cold pattern, one should eat some warm or hot, warming foods.

2. *No matter what, protect and promote the stomach-spleen*

Even though the basic methodology of treatment of Chinese medicine is to administer an "equal opposite" stimulus to bring the person back to balance, no matter what the disease or illness, the process of digestion remains the same. Therefore, the overall requirements for diet also remain the same. Because of the interrelationships between the various viscera and bowels, qi and blood, blood and body fluids, and yin and yang, and because of the pivotal nature of the middle burner or stomach-spleen in the creation and functioning of all of these, adherence to a basic clear, bland, spleen-fortifying diet benefits essentially all conditions.

In other words, one must always be careful when treating any disease with Chinese dietary therapy. Although cold foods are good for a hot disease pattern, one should not eat too many cold and cooling foods. If one does, rather than curing the hot disease pattern, one may only complicate their condition by damaging their stomach-spleen, the source of creation of the healthy or righteous qi which fights disease. If we have a hot pattern, we certainly do not want to eat any hot foods, but we also need to be careful not to eat too many cold and cooling ones. A few carefully selected cold foods which are known to effectively treat the disease at hand in an otherwise level or neutral to slightly warm diet are usually "what the doctor ordered."

Therefore, it is very important to understand that principle number two modifies and moderates principle number one when it comes to remedial Chinese dietary therapy. No matter what the disease, we must protect the stomach-spleen. This is the key to maintaining health and to treating disease. I can't emphasize this too much.

3. *Avoid prohibited foods*

In Chinese dietary therapy, there are certain foods which are prohibited or contraindicated for certain conditions. For instance, slippery, "glossy" foods, such as honey and spinach are contraindicated in cases of slippery, sliding conditions like diarrhea and spermatorrhea.

There is also a whole class of foods which are called *fa wu* in Chinese. The word *fa* means to emit or out-thrust. *Wu* means a material or substance. *Fa wu* foods are those which tend to emit or out-thrust yang qi. In the case of most red-colored skin rashes (which are due to heat), yang qi is already erroneously located and congested in the exterior or the body. If one eats a *fa wu* food, this will only add more yang qi to this heat already congested in the exterior or surface of the body and thus make the skin rash worse. Therefore, *fa wu* foods are prohibited for people who have various types of red skin rashes, such as hives, eczema, psoriasis, and neurodermatitis.

What are some *fa wu* foods? Chicken, shrimp, lobster, clams, mussles, and peanuts are some of the most important and commonly eaten ones. These are foods which are typically hot in nature and supplement liver-kidney yang. Or they are foods which are warm and also dampening and, thus, aggravate damp heat. In any case, one should avoid such *fa wu* foods if they have a hot skin rash. Interestingly, such *fa wu* foods are those which Western medicine considers particularly allergenic.

As the lay reader can see, Chinese dietary therapy can get pretty technical and complicated pretty quickly. Therefore, it is always best to check specific remedial dietary recommendations with a professional TCM practitioner. Nonetheless, there are some general recommendations that can be made regarding the appropriate Chinese dietary therapy for some of the most commonly encountered patterns of imbalance. These are spleen vacuity and dampness, liver depression and stomach heat, kidney yin vacuity, and damp heat.

Spleen Vacuity and Dampness

The spleen may become vacuous or weak due to overfatigue, excessive worry, or overeating sweets and cold, raw foods and drinks. When the spleen becomes weak, its functions of transporting and transforming may become impaired. Typically this results in fluids accumulating in the spleen which are then referred to as pathologic or evil dampness. Once this evil dampness has accumulated in the spleen, it further impairs spleen yang or digestive fire and a vicious circle forms. The spleen is too weak to distill and evaporate or transport and transform this dampness away and this dampness keeps the spleen from recuperating its strength or qi.

This is a commonly encountered problem in clinical practice. Often spleen weakness and dampness begin in infancy with inappropriately scheduled feeding and poor choices in foods for the immature newborn. Spleen weakness and dampness are especially prevalent amongst Westerners. This is because of our current lack of wisdom regarding the feeding of newborns and infants, our sweet tooth, our overconsumption of fats and oils, our use of wheat as our staple grain (which tends to be damp and cool), our fondness for raw, cold, and damp foods in general, too much thinking and worrying, and too little physical exercise. All these factors contribute to the prevalence of spleen weakness and dampness in the West. Because of the pivotal and absolutely crucial importance of stomach-spleen or middle burner function to the health and well-being of the entire organism, such spleen weakness and dampness may cause or complicate innumerable diseases.

If one has been diagnosed by a professional practitioner of TCM as having a weak and/or damp spleen, one should avoid concentrated sweets such as sugar, honey, molasses, and maple syrup. Although some sweets are warm, such as barley malt, and, therefore, not as deleterious to the spleen as, say, white sugar which is cool, still any concentrated sugar can overwhelm the spleen and generate excessive fluids and dampness.

One should minimize their consumption of cold foods. This means foods and drinks which are chilled or frozen. If a food or drink has been stored in the refrigerator, it should be heated up to at least room temperature before being consumed. Person's suffering from spleen weakness and dampness should especially not eat such cold and chilled foods with other foods which would only impair their digestion and absorption. Cold foods also mean energetically cool and cold foods. For instance, lettuce, celery, cucumbers, watermelon, mung beans, buckwheat, seaweed, mango, millet, pears, persimmon, spinach, tomatoes, and wheat are all cool or cold and overconsumption of these foods can chill the middle burner or spleen yang. If these foods are eaten raw or cold, this further worsens their cooling effect.

One should also avoid eating dampening foods and drinking too many liquids with meals. Dampening foods include milk and dairy products, citrus fruits and juices, pineapple juice, tomatoes, sugar and sweets, and fatty, greasy, oily foods. Some persons suffering from spleen dampness may experience constant thirst and may crave liquids. However, this seeming paradox is important to understand. Since fluids are not being transported from the middle burner to the rest of the body in order to moisten and nourish them, these parts of the body may experience thirst or dryness. Yet the more one drinks and floods the spleen with further dampness, the worse and more deeply entrenched this condition becomes. Patients with this diagnosis need to consume less liquids and especially not with meals. At first, their thirst and craving for fluids will increase, but, as the body becomes starved for fluids, the spleen will be forced to give up those that are waterlogging it. Typically, the body's wisdom recognizes what must be done and where to get the liquids it needs within 2-3 days.

What this means from the positive point of view is that people with spleen weakness and dampness should eat a lot of cooked vegetables, cooked rice, small amounts of relatively dry animal protein, such as chicken, turkey, and white fish, and a modicum of preferably cooked fruits. In addition, they should use a moderate amount of drying and warming, spleen strengthening spices and seasonings, such as cardamom, black pepper, ginger (both dry and fresh), cinnamon, and nutmeg. They should eat foods which are light and easy to digest. They should eat soups and stews. And they should chew their food thoroughly. In addition, their practitioners may suggest taking digestive enzymes with meals to supplement their stomach-spleen.

Liver Depression, Stomach Heat

This is another extremely common pattern of imbalance here in the West. Liver depression means stagnation of the qi due to the liver's being jammed up and not free flowing. This is mostly due to emotional stress, what in Chinese is called internal injury due to the seven passions. The Chinese liver is in charge of spreading the qi and maintaining its free flow or patency. Any kind of emotional stress can cause stagnation of liver qi but especially anger and frustration or a feeling of being stuck, trapped, or held back.

Although liver depression and qi stagnation are primarily due to mental/emotional causes, they are complicated by certain dietary factors. The free flow of stomach-spleen qi is dependent in part on the free flow of liver qi. If one overeats and develops food stagnation in the stomach and intestines, this will impede the free flow of stomach-spleen qi which will, in turn, negatively affect liver qi. Therefore, those with liver qi stagnation should be careful not to overeat or stuff themselves full of heavy, hard to digest foods. In other words, one should not eat a lot of nuts, nut butters, bread, and meat.

When the liver becomes stuck, it also becomes full of qi. Since qi is warm, liver stagnation often becomes hot as well. This is called transformative or stagnant heat. Therefore, it is also important not to eat too many energetically hot foods if one's liver tends to be stuck or stagnant. This includes hot, spicy, pungent, and acrid foods. Often people with liver stagnation and depression crave such spicy, hot foods since they are qi stimulants and, at least temporarily, resolve the feeling of impatency and depression. However, if the liver is not only stuck but hot, such hot, spicy foods will cause this heat to flare up even more, thus complicating this scenario. Rather, it is better to increase one's exercise, go to funny movies, practice daily deep relaxation, and attempt to solve those problems in one's life that make one feel stuck and frustrated.

Because the liver and the stomach both get their warmth from the fire of the gate of life, if one of these becomes overheated, the other also typically becomes inflamed. This means that liver depression and stagnant heat are often coupled with a hot stomach as well. Because the liver and gallbladder are a yin/yang pair, if the liver becomes stuck and overheated, the gallbladder can likewise become unhealthily hot. And all this may be compounded by a damp, weak spleen. In such cases, it is important to avoid alcohol, coffee, greasy, oily foods, fatty meats, and chemicals and preservatives. Although one may have an excessive appetite and crave cold foods and drinks, one needs to exercise some care.

If one is truly excess and has a robust spleen but a hot liver and stomach, one's TCM practitioner may advise eating some cold foods, such as raw lettuce, celery, spinach, tofu, soybean sprouts, mung bean sprouts, radishes, coriander, etc. However, that does not mean that these should be overeaten. The middle burner is still the middle burner. One should eat even more freshly cooked vegetables, and especially dark, leafy greens, but one should not go overboard eating all cold, raw foods.

According to the *Nei Jing* (Inner Classic), the foundation classic of Chinese medicine, in cases of liver disease, one should first treat the spleen since, according to five phase theory, the spleen will next be affected if it isn't already. A strong, healthy spleen can do a great deal to keep a full, hot liver in check. Therefore, one should follow the general guidelines for supplementing and disinhibiting the spleen in combination with a modicum of cool and cold foods and medicinals for the liver, gallbladder, and stomach.

Often people with a chronically full and stagnant liver will want to know about the do's and don'ts of diet in great detail. They will gravitate towards lists and stringent and exact guidelines detailing every aspect of what they put in their mouths. This tendency is a symptom of this imbalance. Person's with this complaint should recognize this and try to relax more. Ultimately, liver depression and qi stagnation are emotional issues which need to be addressed primarily on that level. If one with such an imbalance becomes fixated on diet, they miss the point of their diagnosis, for in the end, the key piece of advice to such persons is to kick back and relax.

Kidney Yin Vacuity

Life in the West is extremely fast paced. We are flooded with stimuli, are constantly on the go, and we tend to burn our candles from both ends. Due to sex, drugs, and rock n' roll, many of us have prodigally burnt through our yin substance and *jing* essence. Since the Chinese kidneys are the repository of true or righteous yin and essence, this leads to their weakness and insufficiency. In Chinese medicine, the aging process is exactly equivalent to the weakening and decline of the kidneys. We can say we are as old as our kidneys are. As one ages, one inevitably consumes yin. Thus one becomes dry and wrinkled, stooped and bent, one's hair goes gray or falls out, one's teeth fall, one's vision and hearing become dim, one's sexual capacity declines, and one's mental brilliance begins to fade. TCM attributes all this to kidney weakness and vacuity.

As we have seen in the preceding chapter, the stomach-spleen get the source of their heat from kidney yang or the fire of life. Conversely, the essential substances and nutrients digested by the stomach-spleen are transformed into yin essence which then shore up and bolster the kidneys. In addition, the *Nei Jing* says that the *yang* or stomach and intestinal function begins to decline at around 35, before the kidneys begin their decline.

One of the reasons why many Westerners are prematurely yin empty is that our diet is typically so unsupportive of the stomach-spleen, and the main way to supplement kidney yin dietarily is through strengthening and disinhibiting the spleen. If the spleen is strong and capable of ascending the pure and descending the turbid, an excess of qi and blood is made each day which is converted into essence to be stored in the kidneys when we sleep. Therefore, people with kidney yin emptiness should, once again, eat the basic middle burner benefitting diet described above.

Such patients however, can and should eat a bit more meat and animal proteins than others. Most of the foods which Chinese dietary theory identifies as directly supplementing kidney yin are animal meats and organs. This is because we are talking about yin substance which in the human is one's organs, meat, and flesh. Animal meats and organs are made from the same molecules and constituents as our own body, our own substance. Therefore, such animal foods are the most direct way to get the building blocks and constituents of this yin essence.

Chinese eat all sorts of fish and game that most Westerners do not. Seaslugs, jellyfish, abalone, mussels, clams, testicles, kidneys, hearts, livers, brains, all sorts of eggs, turtles, and all the other fleshy exotica of Chinese cuisine are, from a Chinese medical point of view, eaten because they are kidney yin and essence supplements. However, Chinese doctors also say that these foods should not be overeaten since, because they are so nutritious (*i.e.*, have so much *wei* as compared to qi), they are also dampening, greasy, and hard to digest. Again, the issue is a modicum or moderate amount of these—more perhaps than someone who is not yin empty but not so much as to complicate one's condition with a lot of phlegm and dampness.

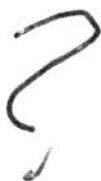

Although lay readers may find it hard at first to understand how a person could be yin vacuous and also damp and phlegmatic (though both are yin, one is righteous and the other is pathologic), many Americans are just that. It is not uncommon in clinical practice to find persons who are damp, phlegmatic, and obese "on the outside" who are parched and dry "on the inside." From a TCM technical point of view, the words inside and outside are not exactly correct, but hopefully one gets the general picture. For these people, sticking to the basic stomach-spleen diet outlined above is their best possible course of action. They should depend upon the connection between the middle burner and the kidneys and the fact that healthy digestion will automatically result in shoring up depleted yin. This was Li Dong-yuan's approach to treating yin vacuity. Li Dong-yuan was one of the four great masters of internal medicine of the Jin-Yuan dynasties (1280-1368 CE).

Therefore, persons with kidney yin vacuity and insufficiency should avoid sugars and sweets, alcohol, coffee, and other stimulants and the excessive use of dry, pungent, warm, and acrid spices. Rather, a person should eat plenty of warm, easy to digest soups and stews, lots of cooked vegetables and grains, and a bit more animal protein than someone else might. As long as a person does not suffer from dampness and phlegm complicating their vacuity and insufficiency, one can eat relatively more wheat and oats which tend to have a lubricating and calming effect.

Damp Heat

The fourth pattern of imbalance which I see most often in clinical practice are various types of damp heat. Most often, the dampness is due to faulty stomach-spleen function. Due to faulty diet, worry, and overfatigue, if the spleen fails to *yun* and *hua* liquids as it should, these, being heavy, have a tendency to seep downwards and collect in the lower part of the body. This dampness impedes the flow of qi wherever it collects. The qi backs up behind the puddled and pooled dampness and, because qi is warm, the area becomes overheated. This heat then becomes tied up or bound with the dampness and becomes what is called in Chinese medicine *shi re* or damp heat. Technically, this heat may be either full, depressive, or empty heat, but, once it joins with dampness, it is damp heat nonetheless.

Damp heat may manifest as problems with the liver and gallbladder or various inflammatory conditions of the intestines, bladder, and reproductive organs. It can also cause various dermatological or skin diseases. Once damp heat gets established in the lower part of the body, it can be difficult to rid. This is due to dampness' heaviness and turbidity. Chinese medicine says dampness is recalcitrant to treatment. In addition, a certain amount of damp heat typically accumulates as one ages.

Since dampness mostly has its source in the middle burner, once again a common sense, middle burner, stomach-spleen benefitting diet is important to correct the generation of dampness at its source. Even if the heat in damp heat is empty heat, such an approach will still benefit the situation. In addition, persons with damp heat in the lower burner or lower half of their body should eat somewhat more cooling, diuretic foods. These include Chinese barley or Job's tears, watermelon and other summer melons, watercress, celery, carrots, cranberries, and cucumbers. However, except for the melons and cranberries, these should all be eaten lightly cooked. Because rice is mildly diuretic, it should be the staple grain for those suffering from damp heat in the lower burner. Sweets, chocolate, nuts, ice cream, frozen yogurt, alcohol, greasy, oily, and fatty foods should be avoided. Chinese dietary theory holds that oils and alcohol are especially productive of dampness and heat.

Neophytes when they first get into Chinese medicine tend to be fascinated by all the exotica. There are any number of Chinese dietary books written in Chinese that give Chinese recipes for various health conditions. It can be fun eating day lily flower because Chinese medicine says these are good for sorrow or turtle and sasparilla soup for damp heat and liver/kidney emptiness. But after more than a dozen years studying, eating, and prescribing Chinese foods according to Chinese dietary theory and therapy, I have come to the conclusion that most people do best if they stick to what I have called a basic middle burner, spleen-benefitting diet: warm food

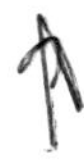

cooked fresh and eaten warm, lots of fresh vegetables, lots of grains, some beans, a little animal protein of all sorts and varieties, a moderate consumption of fruits, seeds, and nuts, not much concentrated sweets, oils, or fats, and plenty of fiber. Professional practitioners or other readers interested in the technical TCM descriptions of specific foods will find these in the rear of this book. However, let me reiterate one more time, I believe it is more important to understand the basic wisdom of Chinese dietary theory than get lost in a sea of technical details and Oriental exotica.

食同藥原 Food Allergies

Food allergies are a common diagnosis amongst Westerners and especially those who seek their health care from so-called alternative practitioners, such as chiropractors, naturopaths, and homeopaths. In Chinese medicine there is no such disease category as food allergies. That is not to say there are no food allergies but that TCM does not categorize the signs and symptoms of such allergies as a distinct disease. In part this is because, in my experience, Chinese are far less prone to food allergies than Westerners. I believe this is so, exactly because traditional Chinese dietary sense is so much better in general than contemporary Western dietary sense. Most Chinese know more about the good and bad effects of food and know better how to eat healthily than most Westerners. Therefore, they have less problems due to eating the wrong foods at the wrong time.

Most food allergies begin in infancy where our current Western lack of nutritional sense is most glaring and apparent. Chinese medical theory states that the child's stomach-spleen or their digestion is immature until at least six years of age. When a person is a beginner at something with undeveloped skills and abilities, we normally recognize the need to start off slowly and easily until one develops the requisite skills and abilities. Babies need to be fed beginner's foods. That means mother's milk, watered down cereal soups, mashed, cooked vegetables, and small amounts of animal soups and broths. Instead, we ply our infants with cold fruit juices, raw carrots, apples, oranges, cheese, fried foods and chips, peanut butter, and cold milk and sweetened yogurt out of the refrigerator.

As we have seen in the preceding chapters, such foods are very dampening and relatively hard to digest. These foods may be very nutritious for a grownup with a strong digestion, but they are very difficult to digest for a child below the age of six. Nonetheless, this is standard fare at most daycare centers and is all too often what our children are given at home. Because these things are damp and hard to digest, they further impair the digestion and tend to cause phlegm and dampness which clog the system. When the flow of qi and blood which are inherently warm get blocked by phlegm and dampness, this heat is transferred to the pathologic accumulations thus causing damp heat and hot phlegm. Most food allergies manifest according to Chinese medicine as some version of heat and/or dampness and phlegm.

It is no wonder then that the foods which are most prone to causing food allergies are those which are the most dampening and phlegmatic. In a study conducted by Dr. Frederic Speer on 1,000 patients, he found that milk, chocolate, cola, corn, citrus, and egg were the most common food allergens. Milk allergies are especially common in children under two. Milk is very dampening according to Chinese dietary theory. Therefore, milk, cheese, and all dairy products tend to aggravate dampness and impede the spleen. If one's digestion is sound, these are very nutritious foods, but it is their very nutritiousness which also causes them to be dampening if one has insufficient spleen qi to distill their dampness.

Chocolate, which is extremely bitter, is rarely eaten alone. It is usually eaten in combination with sugar and tropical, hydrogenated oils.

Chocolate by itself is warm and supplements the *ming men* or fire of life. When eaten with oils and sugars which are extremely dampening, chocolate tends to foster damp heat within the body. Again, this is especially the case with children whose digestion is not capable of transporting and transforming so much dampness and sweets.

Cola is made from a combination of sugars and spices, including cinnamon, citrus, and vanilla. These spices are warm and when eaten with foods are actually digestive aids. However, when taken with sugar water which overwhelms the baby's spleen, they too tend to cause damp heat.

Citrus fruits and juices are sweet and sour. These are the two flavors which in combination tend to be the most dampening according to Chinese five phase theory. Drinking the concentrated essence of oranges, grapefruits, pineapples, and lemons is like mainlining pathogenic dampness. This is especially the case in infants whose yang qi is still struggling to organize and permeate the dampness of their unstructured yin substance.

Corn is sweet with a level or neutral temperature according to Chinese medicine. It is this neutral temperature which makes corn difficult to digest in the newborn besides its tough exterior and the baby's lack of teeth. Because corn lacks its own warmth and yet tends to be dampening because of its sweetness, and since the baby's spleen yang or warmth is weak, this dampness engendered by corn is difficult for the baby to transport and transform.

Eggs are likewise highly nutritious. They have a lot of *wei* as compared to qi. They are a wet, mucousy food which supplements yin and blood. This all adds up to a propensity to be dampening if one's fire of digestion does not burn strongly.

Other foods which cause food allergies and especially in children are soy products. Soybeans are sweet like corn but even cooler. They are quite dampening according to Chinese dietary theory. On the one hand, that makes them nutritious, but, on the other, that makes them hard to digest.

If one is fed or allowed to eat the wrong foods as a child, this can cause chronic spleen dampness and weakness. In Chinese medicine, it is said that dampness is heavy and turbid and hard to resolve. Once pathologic dampness is engendered in the spleen and body as a whole, it is difficult to rid. Therefore, dampness and phlegm engendered as a child may persist into adulthood, especially if one continues to eat the wrong, *i.e.*, damp and difficult to digest, foods. When such foods are eaten, they cause even more dampness and possibly heat and the signs and symptoms of allergy appear.

Although Traditional Chinese Medicine has no category of disease called food allergies, its theory nonetheless explains why certain people experience certain signs and symptoms when they eat certain foods. Allergenic foods almost without exception tend to be dampening and hard to digest.

If one has such a food allergy, it is important to identify the worst offending foods and avoid these. At the same time, a warm, digestion-benefitting diet should be eaten to strengthen the spleen and transform and eliminate chronic dampness. It may take a seemingly long time, but eventually it is possible to strengthen the spleen and eliminate dampness to the point that a moderate amount of the previously allergenic foods can be added back into the diet. However, it should be noted that such highly nutritious, damp-tending foods should not be eaten too frequently nor in too large amounts by anyone. They are immoderate foods which tend to be too yin to eat too much of.

食同藥原 Candidiasis

Many Westerners suffer from candidiasis. Candidiasis is an overgrowth of intestinal yeast. *Candida albicans* are a normal, saprophytic yeast which live in the large intestine and act as scavengers metabolizing debris. However, if they proliferate out of control and if the lining of the intestines becomes too permeable, these yeast can infiltrate and migrate throughout the body. They can cause cystitis and vaginitis, sinusitis, thrush, skin diseases, and a host of other problems. Even if they just stay in the guts, they can cause chronic indigestion, flatulence, constipation or loose stools, fatigue, malaise, and depression.

In addition, overgrowth of *Candida albicans* can cause imbalance in the endocrine system. The endocrine system regulates the hormones and endocrine imbalance can disrupt the menstrual cycle in women causing PMS, early periods, and dysmenorrhea. The endocrine system also regulates the immune system and, therefore, candidiasis can play a very important role in chronic infectious diseases, various viral diseases, and in cancer.

Chinese medicine does recognize the existence of *Candida albicans.* TCM says that this parasite or *chong* in Chinese lives in the intestines and stomach. Further, Chinese medicine believes that it is excessive dampness and heat which provides the environment for run away proliferation of such *chong*. In TCM, candidiasis is always associated with spleen dampness and weakness with a tendency to damp heat.

As we have seen above, dampness is caused by overeating foods which weaken the spleen and engender too much dampness. This includes sugar and refined carbohydrates and citrus fruits and juices. Damp heat *per se* is aggravated by alcohol which is both damp and hot.

Once one has candidiasis, it is important to stay away from eating any foods which tend to be spleen-weakening, damp-engendering, or damp heat-fostering. Also, one should avoid foods contaminated by yeast and fungus. This includes all fermented foods, all yeasted baked good, and anything with vinegar in it. Foods fermented with acidophilus, such as miso, are usually alright. However, because yogurt is made with milk and is, therefore, dampening, it may be contraindicated in certain individuals.

If one has a bad case of candidiasis, fungicidal medicines, whether these be herbal, pharmaceutical, or homeopathic, are often necessary. Some authorities suggest a high protein diet but this may aggravate dampness and heat. Therefore, it is best to eat the basic healthy Chinese maintenance diet described in Chapter 2 but being careful to avoid all yeasted and fermented foods and all dampening, spleen-weakening foods. This means an emphasis on cooked vegetables and complex carbohydrates supplemented by some lean, animal protein.

Other useful books for the lay reader on candidiasis include William G. Crook's *The Yeast Connection* and Trowbridge & Walker's *The Yeast Syndrome.*

食同藥原 Cholesterol

High serum levels of cholesterol have become a national obsession in the United States. Many middle-aged and older Americans consciously attempt to eat a low cholesterol diet. However, the question of cholesterol includes some little understood facts. Although Traditional Chinese Medicine has no concept of cholesterol *per se,* still Western facts regarding cholesterol and diet can be seen through the lens of TCM.

Cholesterol is a nutrient in foods. It is a hormone precursor and so it is found especially in animal foods. Cholesterol is manufactured in our bodies as well as ingested when we eat. Its production is directly related to levels of stress. When we are under stress, our metabolism gears up. The orders for such gearing up are dependent upon hormonal regulation and many important hormones are synthesized from cholesterol. This is evidenced by the fact that many hormones have steroid or sterol in their name, such as the corticosteroids. This is the same sterol as in cholesterol.

The corticosteroids are manufactured in the adrenal cortex sitting on top of the kidneys. These corticosteroids are often referred to as fight or flight hormones. They are the hormones most closely associated with stress reactions in the body. Their manufacture is part of the body's coping mechanism for dealing with stresses of all kinds. What this means is that anything which stresses the body can cause an elevation in cholesterol production as a precursor to producing corticosteroids.

This means that high serum cholesterol levels are not simply a matter of high dietary cholesterol. A person's cholesterol is also a function of their level of stress. Eating sugar, drinking coffee and tea, and drinking alcohol are all stressful to the adrenal glands. From a Chinese medical point of view, coffee, tea, and alcohol liberate a lot of yang qi. Therefore, the body's response is to try to secrete more yin substance. Cholesterol is one such yin substance which becomes pathologic when excessive. Sugar, on the other hand, directly causes the secretion of yin dampness or pathologic substance.

Although eating a diet high in saturated fats can also cause the body to accumulate dampness and phlegm or pathologic yin substance, it is usually not necessary to become fanatical about avoiding all foods containing cholesterol. For instance, eggs have gotten a very bad rap lately because of their high cholesterol content. Chinese medicine believes that eggs are a very nutritious food. Specifically, they are a yin supplement. If a person is able to keep their level of stress under control and avoids sugar, alcohol, coffee, and tea, I believe they can eat a modicum of eggs and certainly more than many people think presently.

I have seen a number of patients with high cholesterol who were on very low cholesterol, restrictive diets and still could not get their cholesterol down. Within weeks after eliminating refined sugars and refined carbohydrates from their diets, all of these patients have been able to reduce their cholesterol levels to within safe limits. At that point, they were able to add back into their diet a modicum of cholesterol-containing foods, such as eggs, and their cholesterol did not increase as long as they avoided sugar.

Therefore, although I agree that one should not eat too many saturated fats, fatty meats, or too many eggs, avoiding sugar and sweets and reducing stress are equally important in maintaining healthy serum cholesterol levels. In TCM terms, cholesterol is a pure yin substance associated with the kidney essence. However, when excessive, it becomes a pathologic yin composed of dampness and phlegm. Therefore, the key to keeping it under healthy control is to keep yang from becoming overly stressed and yin from being overly generated.

食同藥原 Obesity

In Chinese medicine, fat is yin since it is an accumulation of substance. Specifically, TCM holds that fat or adipose tissue is mostly phlegm and dampness. As we have already seen, it is the Chinese spleen which is charged with transportation and transformation of dampness. It is also said in TCM that the spleen is the root of phlegm production. Therefore, Chinese dietary therapy's approach to the treatment of obesity revolves around improving the spleen's transportation and transformation of body fluids and its clean distillation of foods.

As mentioned previously, it is said in the *Nei Jing* that the *yang ming* begins to decline at around the age of 35. The *yang ming* means the stomach and intestines but also can stand for the entire process of digestion including Chinese spleen function. It is a well-known fact that one's metabolism begins to slow down at around 40 and that, even if one eats the same foods and does the same exercise, it is not uncommon to put on 10 pounds or more at that time. The *Nei Jing* also says that in women at around 49 and in men at around 64, the kidneys begin their decline. The kidney fire or the fire of the gate of life is the source of spleen yang or digestive fire. That means that a further gain in weight is also common as the kidneys produce less warmth and, therefore, the body's metabolism or warm transformations slow down even more.

The key to the Chinese dietary treatment of obesity, whether it be lifelong and congenital or due to aging, is to eat easily digestible foods and to keep the fire of digestion as strong and as efficient as possible. That means not eating too many sweet, damp, and greasy, fatty foods. It also means not eating cold foods or drinking cold liquids but rather drinking a small amount of warm liquids with meals. In addition, because the digestion becomes less efficient with age, it becomes all the more important not to overeat and, therefore, jam the qi mechanism.

Regular exercise keeps the qi, blood, and body fluids flowing. As the qi flows, the stomach and intestines conduct the dregs of foods and liquids downward for excretion. It is well known that exercise aids peristalsis and Chinese medical theory supports this fact. Exercise also warms the body up the same way that blowing on a dying fire can rekindle it. Regular, moderate exercise can significantly improve digestion and thus disinhibit the spleen's transportation or circulation of dampness and liquids and the spleens transformation of phlegm or fat. The word transform in Chinese is *hua*. *Hua* also means to melt. It implies a warm transformation. It is interesting to note that we also talk about melting fat away in colloquial English.

New diet programs come and go on a regular basis. Many of them just simply do not work for the majority of people. For instance, drinking copious amounts of cold water before meals in an attempt to fill oneself up only floods the spleen with more dampness. Likewise, drinking large amounts of grapefruit juice only causes the spleen to become damp, sodden, and inefficient. Some of the liquid diet programs currently available and highly touted can be good, but often they include psyllium seeds and oat bran which are both very dampening to the intestines according to Chinese dietary theory. When these are mixed with milk or citrus juices, they can be counterproductive regardless of the number of calories they provide. Although, outside the body, calories are calories, not all foods are digested the same way once inside the body. Professional practitioners of TCM can individually assess each patient's Chinese condition and should be able to tell if a particular diet plan or a particular meal replacement formula is appropriate for a given individual.

Even in Chinese medicine there are wise and less wise ways to go about shedding weight. Within Chinese herbal medicine, there are basically three approaches to weight loss. One approach is to give cold purgatives which essentially chill out the stomach-spleen so that food runs right through one. One loses weight because food is not digested after being eaten. However, since life is warm and since the stomach-spleen are the foundation of the latter heaven or postnatal acquisition of qi and blood, this is a risky approach. It can lead to chronic injury of the stomach-spleen in persons whose stomach-spleens are typically already functioning below par.

A second risky approach is to use pungent, warm, and dry diaphoretics which cause essence to be transformed into qi which is then dispersed upward and outward from the body. In this process, the lungs become hyperactive and discharge fluids and dampness through perspiration and urination. This method is essentially the Chinese equivalent of speed and can cause weakening of the kidneys, exhaustion of essence, and weakening of the lungs. If Olympic athletes use this method and these herbs, notably Herba Ephedrae (the vegetable source of ephedrine), they can be disqualified from their meets. This method is no different or safer than using dexedrin or methamphetamines.

The third approach which, in my opinion, is safer for more people is to use Chinese herbs which benefit digestion and gently seep dampness through increased urination but without causing either drastic purgation of the bowels or exhaustion of essence. Although the first two methods can be used safely by some patients for a limited length of time, they should be administered only on the basis of a professional TCM diagnosis and their use should be monitored continuously. Whereas, the third method of strengthening the spleen, disinhibiting dampness, and transforming phlegm can be safely employed by almost anyone.

It is believed in China that drinking moderate amounts of green tea with meals is very helpful to digestion and can reduce obesity. Green tea is unfermented, whereas black tea is cured and fermented. According to Chinese medicine, green tea strengthens the spleen and disinhibits dampness as well as transforms phlegm. Another helpful, dampness-disinhibiting tea can be made from Job's tears or coix, a Chinese barley. This grain, when taken as a dilute soup or decoction, also strengthens the spleen, disinhibits dampness, promotes drainage of pathologic dampness through urination, and seems to have some preventive ability against cancer.

Therefore, Chinese dietary therapy suggests that those struggling with unwanted weight should eat a diet high in lightly cooked vegetables, high in fiber and complex carbohydrates, mostly warm and easy to digest foods spiced with herbs that aid digestion, and should avoid foods which tend to be damp, phlegmatic, cold, or hard to digest. In addition, one should get more exercise and should consider getting acupuncture or Chinese herbal treatment to strengthen the fire of their digestion. Professional practitioners of Chinese medicine can also usually instruct patients in one or more systems of abdominal self-massage which can likewise stoke the fires of digestion and get the pot of the stomach boiling healthily again.

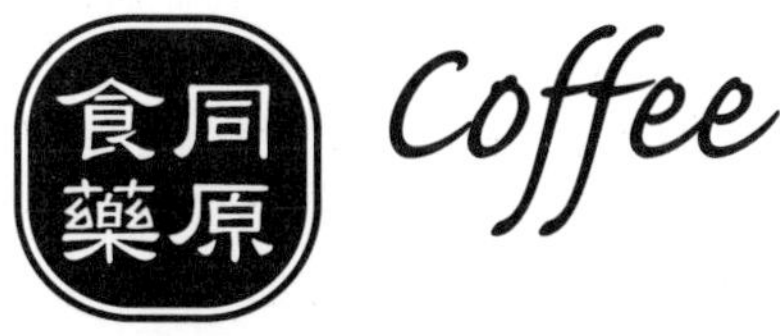

Coffee

In Chinese medicine, coffee is classified as a bitter, pungent, and warm exterior-resolving medicinal. Exterior-resolvers are basically diaphoretics. These medicinals work by transforming kidney yin or essence into qi which is then liberated upward and outward through the system. As these move outward through the body's various energetic layers, they flood the organs within these layers with yang qi and so one experiences increased energy. In addition, this yang qi moving upward and outward promotes the flow of all the qi of the body, liberating stuck qi and with it activating blood and body fluids.

People who are either producing less qi from their daily diet, are using more qi through hyperactivity than they make each day, fail to store the qi they make because of disturbed sleep, or who lack access to their qi because of its being bound up or stagnant will all experience temporary access to abundant qi and the sense of energy and flow that go along with that when they drink coffee. However, because coffee is warm by nature, it tends to heat the stomach. This results in coffee's causing hot loose stools in many people with an attendant loss of spleen qi. Because coffee stimulates the lungs' participation in the downward transportation of body fluids to the bladder, it is also a diuretic. Each time we urinate, we lose qi since urine does not just dribble out but is transported. This means that we also lose warmth since qi is yang and, therefore, warm. Such diuresis weakens kidney yang at the same time as coffee steals kidney yin or essence.

Coffee, therefore, has a debilitating effect on both the middle and lower burners. Spleen qi is lost and kidney yin and yang are exhausted. Using coffee as an energy boost is like continually dipping into one's savings or capital. Eventually such profligate deficit spending leaves one's internal economy bankrupt. When coffee transforms and liberates essence qi, one gets a rush but ultimately loses that precious stored energy.

When coffee was first introduced into Europe, there were prohibition movements and laws based on the recognition that coffee is a powerful and not wholly benign drug. Although coffee has certain legitimate medical and emergency uses, its use as a daily beverage is not very wise. It is my belief that if coffee were to be introduced to the West today as a new discovery, governmental agencies, such as the FDA in the United States, would restrict its use as a controlled substance. Since the government of the United States cannot, due to economic pressures, outlaw cigarette smoking which has incontestably been shown to be linked to lung cancer, it is even less likely that this common beverage could be prohibited at this late date. However, except as a medicinal and in cases where the use of speed is warranted knowing full well the risks its use entails, I believe coffee has no place in the diet of those hoping to be healthy. It is one of the few foods that I unequivocally deny to my patients.

Women especially do well to avoid coffee. Because of the violent upward dispersal coffee initiates in the body, it seems to injure the *chong mai*. The *chong mai* is an energy pathway running up the very core of the body connecting the kidneys to the heart. The purpose of this pathway is to feed kidney yang to the heart where it is transformed into the light of consciousness or *shen ming.* It also leads kidney yin upwards to provide the nourishment and substantial support for the "higher" activities of consciousness and sensation. In injuring this connection between above and below, heart and kidneys, and exhausting yin, blood, and righteous body fluids, coffee tends to cause accumulations in women's breasts above and in their pelvises below. Although controlled tests have so far not confirmed this fact, their results are, in my opinion, due to a flaw in their design and logic, since every astute clinician knows from experience that coffee negatively affects women's breasts and reproductive organs.

食同
藥原

Vitamins

When I first began practicing TCM or Chinese medicine, I, like most converts to a new belief system, strove to hew to a very pure, traditional Chinese practice. I perceived things like Western vitamin and mineral supplements as incompatible with such a pure, traditional approach. This was in the face of the fact that Chinese practitioners of TCM do not have any problem with using vitamin and mineral supplements. At that time, I confused Chinese medicine as a system of thought with medicines which come from China. These are not necessarily the same thing.

In Chinese medicine, probably as much as 20% of the standard repertoire of 500 medicinal substances originated outside of China. Spices such as cardamon, cloves, nutmeg, and cinnamon came from southeast and southwest Asia and the Spice Islands. Apricot, peach, and prune pits came from Central Asia and the Mideast. Licorice came from southern Russia. Cinchona bark came from the Andes. Eagleswood, saffron, and terminalia came from India and the Himalayas. And American ginseng and greater celandine came from the United States and Canada.

In addition, Chinese medicinals, although referred to even in Chinese as *yao* or herbs, are not all herbal in origin. Rather they come from all three kingdoms—animal, vegetable, and mineral. Further, Chinese doctors did not and do not only use naturally occurring medicinal substances found in their raw form. Chinese doctors and pharmacists have for centuries studied and employed a host of processing and refining techniques in order to make their medicinals more powerful and concentrated with less side effects and toxicity. So-called Chinese herbal medicine was largely the product of Daoist alchemists who were also the progenitors of the science of chemistry.

Therefore, there is no Chinese precedent for thinking that a practitioner of so-called Chinese medicine must only prescribe medicinals which originate in China, medicinals originating from vegetable or herbal sources, or naturally occurring substances in their raw or unprocessed form. That means there is no *a priori* reason vitamins and minerals cannot be incorporated into the contemporary practice of Traditional Chinese Medicine.

When vitamins, minerals, amino acids, enzymes, coenzymes, fatty acids, and cofactors are used medicinally, these are referred to as orthomolecular supplements. Orthomolecular means the same molecules as the body itself. Orthomolecular supplements are essentially concentrations of nutrient substances normally found in the foods we eat. Many people ask, if vitamins and minerals are simply found in the foods we eat, why can't we get enough of these in our daily diet? That is a good question but one which can be easily answered.

First of all, many people in the West do not eat a healthy and balanced diet. We tend not to eat enough fresh vegetables and we tend to eat too much sugar, protein, and fats. These foods cause us to use up inordinate amounts of certain other nutrients. For instance, if one eats lots of meat, one needs more calcium. And sugar causes us to use up more zinc.

Secondly, many of the foods we eat are grown in poor soil due to excessive use of chemical fertilizers and other modern but short-sighted farming practices. This is compounded by the fact that many people today eat foods which have been prepared and stored by canning, freezing, and dehydrating which cause some loss of vitamins and enzymes.

Third, we are exposed to toxic chemicals in our air, water, and food which are a type of extra stress on our systems requiring extra nutrients to neutralize these.

Fourth, most of us living in urban environments are subject to large amounts of mental and emotional stress. It is my belief that simply living in the urban West is more than our nervous systems are capable of dealing with in a healthy way. There are just too many and unrelieved stresses which are constantly assaulting us. Such stress uses up inordinate amounts of B vitamins and minerals.

Fifth, if one drinks coffee or alcohol, smokes cigarettes, is exposed to radiation, is taking certain medications, such as oral birth control pills, or is suffering from a chronic illness, and especially a digestive complaint, any one of these is using up abnormally large amounts of certain nutrients or is not absorbing others from their food.

For all these reasons, one may need to supplement certain nutrients which are not adequately found in their diet. This does not mean that if one gobbles lots of vitamins one does not need to eat a healthy diet. What it does mean is that, given the stressful, polluted world we live in, we may not be getting enough vital nutrients simply from our diet.

Over the last seven or eight years, I have attempted to develop preliminary TCM descriptions of all the common vitamins, minerals, and amino acids. Using these descriptions, Western practitioners of TCM might prescribe orthomolecular supplements based on a TCM diagnosis just as if they were prescribing Chinese herbs. Although this is not something I suggest laypersons do for themselves, I have included this brief discussion of orthomolecular supplements in this layperson's guide to Chinese dietary therapy primarily to let patients know that such supplements are consistent with the practice of TCM. They are a useful adjunct to other, more standard TCM therapies and should not be overlooked simply because they are not "Chinese." These descriptions emphasize that TCM is more a system of thinking about health and disease than a collection of exotic treatments from the Far East.

TCM Functions of Vitamins

Vitamin A: Supplements the blood and fills the essence, brightens the eyes and clears heat from the blood; treats vacuity heat patterns.

Vitamin B_1: Courses the liver and rectifies the qi, fortifies the spleen and dries dampness, stops pain.

Vitamin B_2: Nourishes the liver and supplements the kidneys, engenders fluids and boosts the stomach.

Vitamin B_3: Soothes the liver and harmonizes the stomach, fortifies the spleen and clears heat from the stomach, upbears the clear and frees the flow of the qi mechanism.

Vitamin B_5: Courses the liver and rectifies the qi, clears heat and resolves depression, supplements the spleen and harmonizes the stomach.

Vitamin B_6: Courses the liver and rectifies the qi, clears heat and resolves depression, harmonizes wood and earth, clears heat from the stomach and damp heat from the gallbladder.

Vitamin B_{12}: Supplements the qi and nourishes the blood, stops bleeding.

Vitamin B_{15}: Rectifies and moves the qi, quickens the blood and transforms stasis.

Biotin: Nourishes the blood and emolliates the liver, supplements the heart and quiets the spirit.

Choline: Nourishes the blood and extinguishes wind, strengthens the sinews and bones, moistens the intestines and frees the flow of the stool.

Folic acid: Nourishes the blood and harmonizes the liver, quiets the spirit and the fetus.

Inositol: Nourishes the blood, moistens the intestines, and quiets the spirit.

PABA: Supplements the liver and kidneys, moistens the intestines and frees the flow of the stool, dispels wind, blackens the hair, and retards aging.

Vitamin C: Clears heat and stops bleeding, clears heat and resolves toxins, clears heat from the heart and quiets the spirit.

Vitamin D: Supplements the kidneys and invigorates yang, strengthens the sinews and bones, brightens the eyes and quiets the fetus.

Vitamin E: Nourishes the blood and supplements yang, strengthens the sinews and bones.

Vitamin K: Secures and astringes the lungs and large intestine, stops bleeding.

Bioflavonoids: Clears heat from the blood and stops bleeding, quickens the blood and transforms stasis.

Beta-carotene: Courses the liver and rectifies the qi, clears heat and resolves toxins, disperses stagnations and accumulations, combats cancer.

TCM Functions of Minerals

Calcium: Astringes yin and suppresses yang, strengthens the bones and promotes the generation of new tissue, absorbs acid and stops pain.

Chromium: Fortifies the spleen and boosts the qi, supplements the qi and blood.

Cobalt: Supplements the qi to transform blood.

Copper: Fortifies the spleen and seeps dampness, clears and eliminates damp heat.

Flourine: Supplements the kidneys and enriches yin, strengthens the bones and teeth.

Iodine: Courses the liver and rectifies the qi, clears heat and scatters nodulation.

Iron: Clears heat and cools the blood, quickens the blood and transforms stasis.

Magnesium: Astringes yin and suppresses yang, quiets the spirit, absorbs acid, and stops pain.

Manganese: Nourishes the liver and enriches the kidneys, strengthens the sinews and bones, sharpens the hearing.

Molybdenum: Nourishes the blood and enriches yin, clears heat and cools the blood.

Phosphorus: Supplements the kidneys and enriches yin, strengthens the sinews and bones.

Potassium: Fortifies the spleen and seeps dampness, clears heat and expels pus, dispels wind dampness, clears and eliminates damp heat.

Selenium: Astringes yin and suppresses yang, quiets the spirit and brightens the eyes.

Silica: Supplements the kidneys and strengthens the bones.

Silicon: Supplements the liver and kidneys and strengthens the sinews and bones.

Sodium: Supplements the liver and kidneys and secures the essence, softens hardness and scatters nodulation.

Sulfur: Supplements the kidneys and warms yang, blackens the hair and benefits the skin.

Zinc: Nourishes the liver and enriches the kidneys, strengthens the bones and brightens the eyes.

TCM Functions of Amino Acids

Alanine: Fortifies the spleen and boosts the qi, nourishes the heart and quiets the spirit.

Arginine: Supplements the kidneys and invigorates yang, moistens the intestines and frees the flow of the stool, strengthens the sinews and bones and dispels wind cold dampness.

BCAA (Leucine, Isoleucine & Valine): Supplements the kidneys and enriches yin.

Carnitine: Supplements the blood and yin.

Cysteine: Nourishes the liver and enriches the kidneys, clears heat and cools the blood, clears heat and resolves toxins, blackens the hair and promotes the generation of new tissue.

Glutamic acid: Supplements the kidneys and enriches yin.

Glutathione: Clears heat and resolves toxins, clears heat and cools the blood, promotes lactation.

Glycine: Supplements the blood and promotes the growth of new tissue.

Histidine: Supplements the blood and yin, may clear heat and cool the blood.

Lysine: Supplements the blood and yin, may clear heat and resolve toxins.

Methionine: Nourishes and cools the blood, soothes the liver and quiets the spirit.

Ornithine: Supplements yang.

Phenyalinine: Resolves the exterior and clears heat, clears heat and resolves toxins, moves the qi and stops pain.

Taurine: Clears heat and resolves toxins, drains the liver and clears damp heat from the gallbladder, promotes lactation.

Threonine: Nourishes the blood and extinguishes wind, soothes the liver and relieves tension and contractions.

Tryptophan: Courses the liver and resolves depression, quickens the blood and transforms stasis, quiets the spirit and stops pain.

Tyrosine: Courses the liver and rectifies the qi, harmonizes wood and earth.

Because the basic methodology of Chinese medicine is to prescribe the equal opposite force necessary to bring a person back into healthy balance, if one knows that they are too hot, then taking vitamin C makes perfect sense according to the logic of TCM. Conversely, because vitamin C is cold and clears heat, taking too much of it can damage the spleen and lead to spleen vacuity loose stools and diarrhea. In the same way, one can decide on who should take what amounts of the above vitamins, minerals, and amino acids.

Because, vitamin and mineral supplements provide very concentrated doses of these ingredients, I believe they should be regarded as medicinals rather than as foods. This means that they should be prescribed with the same care and thought as any other medicinal, be that a Chinese herb or Western pharmaceutical. If something is strong enough to bring a person back to balance when necessary, then that same thing must also be strong enough to push a person out of balance when unnecessary or inappropriate. You can't have it both ways. So the stronger a medicinal is, the more care should be exercised in its choice and use.

The beauty of Chinese medicine is that, using its system of prescribing, one can tell exactly who needs what medicines in what amounts. Thus Chinese medicine, when correctly practiced, provides healing without side effects. Each person gets just the right treatment for their individual needs. This is exactly what makes TCM the safe and effective system of medicine it is and why it provides such a wonderful alternative and complement to modern Western medicine which tends to prescribe the same medicine for all persons with the same disease. Since each person is different from every other person, no one medicine, or nutritional supplement is going to be right for every person even with the same disease. And that is why one gets side effects.

As an extension of this, just as one can work out the Chinese medical descriptions of Western orthomolecular supplements, one can also work out the descriptions of Western pharmaceuticals which then could also be prescribed without side effects.

食同 藥原 TCM Descriptions of Commonly Eaten Foods

Below are the Chinese medical descriptions of more than 150 commonly eaten foods. These descriptions are all taken from Chinese sources. However, they are also all foods which are found and eaten in the West. They are found in either grocery stores, health food stores, Asian specialty food shops, or, in a few instances, in your backyard. The categories of information under each food are flavor, nature or temperature, channel entering, functions or actions, and indications.

In Chinese medicine, there are six flavors: sweet, salty, sour, acrid, bitter, and bland. The flavors of each food are based on direct sensory experience, and many if not most foods are combinations of more than a single flavor. Of these six flavors, five correspond with five phase theory and each "enters" one of the five main viscera of Chinese medicine. Sweet enters the spleen. Sour enters the liver. Bitter enters the heart. Acrid enters the lungs. And salty enters the kidneys. In small amounts, these flavors benefit these viscera but, in large amounts, they actually damage them. In addition, each of the six flavors tends to have certain effects on the body. The sweet flavor boosts the qi and engenders fluids. The bitter flavor tends to astringe and dry as well as lead the qi downward. The sour flavor also astringes and constrains. The acrid flavor leads the qi upward and outward and tends to also be drying, while the salty flavor leads the qi downward and softens hardness. The bland flavor also leads downward and promotes urination. Therefore, by knowing the flavor of a food, we can know a lot about the viscera it may enter and the effects it may have on the body.

Likewise, herbs and foods can have five natures or temperatures: cold, cool, level (*i.e.*, balanced or neutral), warm, and hot. These natures, also sometimes referred to as a food's qi, describe the effect of the food on the body's temperature. In other words, warm and hot foods tend to heat the body up, while cool and cold foods tend to cool the body down. These descriptions are more theoretical than a food's flavor, and so are open to more differences of opinion in the Chinese medical literature. It is not uncommon to find one author who says a food is level, while another says it is cool or warm. Happily, such differences of opinion are usually never so great as to be completely opposite—one authority saying a food is hot while another saying it's cold. These temperatures have been worked out by Chinese medical thinkers based on the conditions a given food benefits and whether Chinese medicine defines those conditions as hot or cold. In other words, a food is usually considered cold if all the diseases or patterns it treats are hot.

Channel enterings describe which viscera or bowel a food exerts its most pronounced influences on. Although the Chinese words are *gui jing*, channel gathering, these influences are not on the channels *per se* but rather on the organs. This information is even more theoretical than a food's nature. It is a relatively late addition to Chinese medical theory (beginning in the 12th century) and was definitely arrived at by working backwards from the conditions a food treats to the main viscera and bowels associated with that condition. Because of the many differences of opinion about these channel enterings, many Chinese dietary manuals leave out this information altogether, and, in any case, the reader should take it "with a grain of salt."

Functions refer to the actions of a food on the body stated in terms of TCM theory. These functions describe how a food exerts the healing influences on the body that it does. In other words, if a food is said to clear heat and eliminate dampness and this is then followed by the fact that it is used to treat cholecystitis, then we know that it specifically treats damp heat in the gallbladder and that it restores balance and health to the body by getting rid of pathological heat and somehow eliminating too much dampness. In Chinese medical texts, these functions are also referred to as treatment principles when they are used in terms of treating disease. In that case, such treatment principles are the bridge or link which allows one to go from the TCM pattern discrimination to the choice of remedies. For instance, cholecystitis may also be due to liver depression and blood stasis. In that case, we still need a food or herb which treats cholecystitis, but now we need one which courses the liver and rectifies the qi, quickens the blood and transforms stasis. Therefore, these functions (and treatment principles) are extremely important to the proper practice of TCM.

Indications refer to the symptoms, conditions, or diseases a food is known to treat based on real-life, clinical experience. In theory, a certain food with a certain nature, flavor, and functions should be able to treat this or that disease, but in fact, it may not. Therefore, the Chinese medical description of each food is a combination of finely honed theory and centuries of direct observation. These two, theory and practice, are the two wings of the bird of medicine. As Albert Einstein once said, "Theory without practice is sterile, but practice without theory is blind." With both these wings working in coordination, the bird of medicine can fly to heaven!

Therefore, the reader should take care not to grab at only a part of any food's Chinese medical description. You have to take the whole description into account and then think about it a bit. For instance, sugar is said to be sweet and boosts the qi. However, it also engenders fluids. While we may all think more qi or energy is good, eating too much sugar will actually generate too much dampness in the body. Likewise, we may find a food that is listed for a disease we have and think that we should eat a lot of it. However, if its nature, flavor, and functions do not match our individual TCM pattern, this food is not going to do us much good and may actually do us harm.

Not every food we Westerners eat is found on this list. One of the outcomes of Columbus's "discovery" of the New World was a huge explosion in the numbers of varieties of foods. Chinese doctors have not had the time or opportunity to work out the Chinese medical descriptions of all of these. For instance, the reader will find peanuts, pine nuts, and almonds on the list below, but there is no Chinese medical descriptions of cashews and Brazil nuts. In this case, we know that all unsalted nuts are primarily sweet and all contain lots of oil. This means that all nuts are highly nutritious and contain a lot of *wei* or flavor. In small amounts, they supplement vacuity and moisten dryness. But overeaten or eaten by a person with spleen vacuity weakness, they may engender dampness and phlegm. Similarly, we can know something about nectarines by comparing them with peaches and plums. Both are at least partially sweet and both engender fluids. Therefore, people with spleen dampness probably should take care when it comes to nectarines. In other words, even though a food may be missing from this list, we should be able to work out at least some of its Chinese medical description if we think about similar foods in its class and their TCM descriptions.

Abalone
Nature, flavor & channel entering: Sweet, salty, and level; enters the liver and kidney channels.

Functions & indications: Enriches yin and clears heat, fills the essence and brightens the eyes; treats dry cough, vaginal discharge, vaginal bleeding, urinary strangury, and cataracts.

Aduki bean
Nature, flavor & channel entering: Sweet, sour, and level; enters the heart and small intestine channels.

Functions & indications: Clears heat and disinhibits urination, quickens the blood and transforms stasis, drains fire and resolves toxins; treats edema, leg qi, inhibited urination, sores, hemorrhoidal bleeding, and mild jaundice.

Agar
Nature, flavor & channel entering: Sweet and cold; enters the lung and large intestine channels.

Functions & indications: Clears heat in the lungs and upper burner; treats cough and hemorrhoids.

Alcohol
Nature, flavor & channel entering: Bitter, sweet, acrid, warm, and toxic; enters the heart, liver, lung, and stomach channels.

Functions & indications: Frees the flow of the blood vessels and disperses cold qi, arouses the spleen and warms the stomach; treats wind cold impediment pain, contracture and spasm of the sinews and vessels, chest impediment, and chilly pain in the heart and abdomen.

Alfalfa sprout
Nature, flavor & channel entering: Bitter and cool; enters the spleen, stomach, and large intestine channels.

Functions & indications: Dries dampness, clears heat from the spleen and stomach, frees urination and defecation, expels stones; treats urinary stones and edema and heat accumulation constipation.

Almond

Nature, flavor & channel entering: Sweet and level; enters the lung and large intestine channels.

Functions & indications: Moistens the lungs, levels panting, and frees the flow of the stool; treats vacuity taxation coughing and panting and intestinal dryness constipation.

Anise

Nature, flavor & channel entering: Acrid, sweet, and warm; enters the spleen, kidney, and liver channels.

Functions & indications: Warms yang and moves the qi; treats constipation, difficult urination, abdominal distention, mounting pain, and low back pain.

Apple

Nature, flavor & channel entering: Sweet and cool; enters the lung, stomach, and large intestine channels.

Functions & indications: Engenders fluids and moistens the lungs, eliminates vexation and resolves summerheat, opens the stomach and arouses from alcohol.

Apricot

Nature, flavor & channel entering: Sweet, sour, and level; enters the spleen, stomach, lungs, and large intestine channels.

Functions & indications: Moistens the lungs, levels panting, engenders fluids and relieves thirst; treats dry throat, dry cough, thirst, and fluid dryness constipation.

Asparagus

Nature, flavor & channel entering: Sweet, bitter, and cold; enters the lung, spleen, and kidney channels.

Functions & indications: Clears heat and eliminates dampness, moistens dryness and clears the lungs; treats hemoptysis, enduring cough, wasting thirst, and constipation.

Bamboo shoot

Nature, flavor & channel entering: Sweet and cold; enters the large intestine, lung, and stomach channels.

Functions & indications: Clears heat and transforms phlegm, harmonizes the center and moistens the intestines; treats phlegm heat congestion and exuberance, food distention, non-easy defecation, and non-emission of measles rash.

Banana

Nature, flavor & channel entering: Sweet and cool; enters the lungs and large intestine channels.

Functions & indications: Clears heat, moistens the intestines, and resolves toxins; treats heat diseases, vexatious thirst, and hemorrhoidal bleeding.

Barley

Nature, flavor & channel entering: Sweet, salty, and slightly cold; enters the spleen, stomach, and gallbladder channels.

Functions & indications: Clears heat and eliminates dampness, boosts the qi and regulates the center, cools the blood and transforms accumulations, strengthens the force (*i.e.*, physical strength) and nourishes the blood, fortifies the spleen and disinhibits urination; treats indigestion, diarrhea, edema, and jaundice.

Basil

Nature, flavor & channel entering: Acrid and warm; enters the lung, spleen, stomach, and large intestine channels.

Functions & indications: Rectifies the qi and blood, scatters cold, dispels wind and eliminates dampness, and resolves toxins; treats external pattern headache, abdominal distention and pain, menstrual irregularities, diarrhea, and burping and belching.

Beef

Nature, flavor & channel entering: Sweet and level; enters the spleen, liver, kidneys, stomach, and large intestine channels.

Functions & indications: Supplements the qi and blood, enriches yin and engenders fluids, strengthens the sinews and bones; treats emaciation and cachexia, edema, wasting thirst, yin vacuity low back and knee pain and weakness.

Beet

Nature, flavor & channel entering: Sweet and level or cooling; enters the heart and liver channels.

Functions & indications: Nourishes and quickens the blood, supplements the heart and clears the liver, moistens the intestines; treats menstrual irregularities, blood vacuity, and fluid dryness constipation.

Black fungus (a.k.a. tree ears)

Nature, flavor & channel entering: Sweet and level; enters the stomach and large intestine channels.

Functions & indications: Cools and quickens the blood and stops bleeding; treats blood stasis after external injury and childbirth, bleeding hemorrhoids, and vaginal bleeding.

Black pepper

Nature, flavor & channel entering: Acrid and hot; enters the stomach and large intestine channels.

Functions & indications: Warms the center and descends the qi, disperses phlegm and resolves toxins; treats cold phlegm, food accumulation, epigastric chilly pain, hiccup, vomiting of clear water, diarrhea, and chilly dysentery.

Broccoli

Nature, flavor & channel entering: Sweet, slightly bitter, and cool; enters the spleen, stomach, and bladder channels.

Functions & indications: Clears heat and disinhibits urination, brightens the eyes and resolves summerheat; treats red, painful eyes, difficult urination, and vexatious heat.

Buckwheat

Nature, flavor & channel entering: Sweet and cool; enters the spleen, stomach, and large intestine channels.

Functions & indications: Opens the stomach and loosens the intestines, descends the qi and disperses accumulations; treats intestine and stomach accumulation and stagnation, chronic diarrhea, dysentery prohibiting eating, welling and flat abscesses on the upper back, scrofulas, and scalding burns.

Burdock root

Nature, flavor & channel entering: Acrid, bitter, and slightly cold; enters the liver and stomach channels.

Functions & indications: Clears heat and resolves toxins, combats cancer; treats various sorts of malign and toxic sores.

Cabbage
Nature, flavor & channel entering: Sweet, slightly bitter, and cool; enters the spleen, stomach, and large intestine channels.

Functions & indications: Clears the blood and fortifies the stomach, disinhibits the intestines and frees the flow of the stool, eliminates vexation within the chest, and resolves alcoholic thirst; treats constipation in the elderly and in women.

Cantaloupe (honeydew, muskmelon, etc.)
Nature, flavor & channel entering: Sweet, aromatic, and cool; enters the lungs, heart, large intestine, small intestine, and bladder channels.

Functions & indications: Clears heat, moistens the lungs, and disinhibits urination; treats fever with thirst, reddish, scanty urination, dry cough, and fluid dryness constipation.

Carambola (a.k.a. star fruit)
Nature, flavor & channel entering: Sour, sweet, and level; enters the spleen, stomach, lungs, large intestine, and bladder channels.

Functions & indications: Engenders fluids and stops cough, downbears upward counterflow and harmonizes the stomach; treats sore throat, sores in the mouth, wind heat toothache and cough, hiccup, nausea, and indigestion, red, scanty, painful urination, hematuria, urticaria, and pruritus.

Caraway seed
Nature, flavor & channel entering: Slightly acrid and warm; enters the liver, kidney, and stomach channels.

Functions & indications: Moves the qi and opens the stomach, courses the liver and warms the kidneys; treats indigestion, abdominal distention, nausea, hiccup, scanty appetite, vomiting, mounting pain, and cold menstrual pain.

Cardamon
Nature, flavor & channel entering: Acrid, aromatic, and warm; enters the spleen and stomach channels.

Functions & indications: Transforms dampness and stops vomiting, rectifies the qi and harmonizes the stomach, quiets the fetus; treats nausea, vomiting, indigestion, abdominal distention and pain, loss of appetite, diarrhea, nausea during pregnancy, and threatened miscarriage.

Carrot
Nature, flavor & channel entering: Sweet, acrid, and level or slightly warm; enters the lung and spleen channels.

Functions & indications: Fortifies the spleen and transforms stagnation; treats indigestion, enduring dysentery, and cough.

Cauliflower
Nature, flavor & channel entering: Sweet, slightly bitter, and slightly warm; enters the spleen and stomach channels.

Functions & indications: Fortifies the spleen, scatters cold, and stops pain; treats indigestion.

Cayenne pepper
Nature, flavor & channel entering: Acrid and hot; enters the spleen and stomach channels.

Functions & indications: Dispels cold and fortifies the stomach, quickens the blood and moves the qi; treats indigestion, loss of appetite, and wind damp cold impediment.

Celery
Nature, flavor & channel entering: Sweet, bitter, and cool; enters the stomach and liver channels.

Functions & indications: Levels the liver and clears heat, dispels wind and disinhibits dampness; treats high blood pressure, dizziness and vertigo, headache, red face and red eyes, bloody dysentery, and welling abscesses and swellings.

Cherry

Nature, flavor & channel entering: Sweet, aromatic, and warm; enters the spleen, stomach, lung, heart, and kidney channels.

Functions & indications: Supplements the qi, nourishes the blood, and engenders fluids, quickens the blood and transforms stasis, dispels wind dampness; treats wind heat dryness sore throat, qi and blood vacuity weakness, wind damp impediment in the lower half of the body, and numbness and paraylsis.

Chestnut

Nature, flavor & channel entering: Sweet and warm; enters the spleen, stomach, and kidney channels.

Functions & indications: Nourishes the stomach and fortifies the spleen, supplements the kidneys and strengthens the sinews, quickens the blood and stops bleeding; treats spleen-stomach vacuity weakness, nausea, diarrhea, constitutional vacuity low back soreness and lower leg weakness, epistaxis, hematemesis, hemafecia, metal wounds, contusions causing swelling and pain, scrofulas, and swelling toxins.

Chicken

Nature, flavor & channel entering: Sweet and warm; enters the spleen, stomach, and kidney channels.

Functions & indications: Supplements the qi and blood, warms the internal, and invigorates the kidneys; treats poor appetite, diarrhea, edema, frequent urination, vaginal bleeding and vaginal discharge, scanty lactation, and fatigue.

Chicken egg
Nature, flavor & channel entering: Sweet and level; enters the five viscera and stomach.

Functions & indications: Nourishes the blood and enriches yin, brightens the eyes and moistens dryness; treats dry cough, dry, sore throat, hoarse voice, blurred vision, and various blood vacuity-yin insufficiency conditions.

Chive
Nature, flavor & channel entering: Acrid and warm; enters the liver, kidney, and stomach channels.

Functions & indications: Rectifies the qi and blood, scatters cold and harmonizes the stomach; treats blood stasis due to traumatic injury, indigestion, abdominal distention, scanty appetite, nausea, and vomiting due to stomach cold.

Cinnamon
Nature, flavor & channel entering: Acrid, sweet, and hot; enters the kidney, spleen, and bladder channels.

Functions & indications: Supplements the source yang, warms the spleen and stomach, eliminates accumulation and chill, and frees the flow of the blood vessels; treats life gate fire debility, chilled limbs, a faint pulse, collapse of yang, vacuity desertion, abdominal pain, diarrhea, cold mounting, low back and knee chilly pain, blocked menstruation, concretions and conglomerations, weeping yin flat abscesses, and heat above but cold below due to upward floating of vacuous yang.

Clam
Nature, flavor & channel entering: Salty, sweet, and cold; enters the spleen and stomach, liver and kidney channels.

Functions & indications: Frees the flow of the water passageways, transforms phlegm and softens hardness, supplements the liver and kidneys; treats edema, profuse phlegm, goiter, lymphadenopathy, vaginal discharge, dry cough, and night sweats.

Cloves

Nature, flavor & channel entering: Acrid and warm; enters the kidney, spleen, and stomach channels.

Functions & indications: Warms the center and downbears upwardly counterflow qi, warms the kidneys and invigorates yang; treats stomach cold vomiting, hiccup, abdominal pain and diarrhea, clear, chilly vaginal discharge, cold uterus infertility, and yang vacuity impotence.

Coconut

Nature, flavor & channel entering: Sweet and warm; enters the spleen, stomach, and large intestine channels.

Functions & indications: Engenders fluids, disinhibits urination, and expels worms; treats vexatious thirst, wasting thirst, severe dehydration after bleeding or severe diarrhea, edema, and tapeworm and fascioliasis.

Coffee

Nature, flavor & channel entering: Bitter, acrid, and warm; enters the lung, liver, kidney, and stomach channels.

Functions & indications: Moves the qi and quickens the blood, resolves the exterior and disinhibits urination; treats chronic bronchitis, emphysema, *cor pulmonale*, and hangover from alcohol.

Coriander

Nature, flavor & channel entering: Acrid and warm; enters the lung and spleen channels.

Functions & indications: Emits sweat and out-thrusts rashes, disperses food and descends the qi; treats measles which are not easily out-thrust, and food accumulation and stagnation.

Corn

Nature, flavor & channel entering: Sweet and level; enters the heart, lung, spleen, liver, stomach, gallbladder, and bladder channels.

Functions & indications: Boosts the lungs and settles the heart, regulates the center and opens the stomach, disinhibits urination and the gallbladder; treats difficult urination, gallstones, jaundice, hepatitis, and hypertension.

Crab

Nature, flavor & channel entering: Salty and cold; enters the liver and stomach channels.

Functions & indications: Clears heat, scatters the blood, and promotes the union of broken bones; treats detriment damage to the sinews and bones, scabies, lacquer dermatitis, and scalding burns (when applied externally).

Crayfish (including lobster)

Nature, flavor & channel entering: Sweet, salty, and warm; enters the liver and kidney channels.

Functions & indications: Supplements the kidneys and boosts yang; treats sinew and bone pain and hemiplegia after an attack of phlegm fire (*i.e.*, stroke).

Dill

Nature, flavor & channel entering: Acrid and warm; enters the spleen, kidney, and stomach channels.

Functions & indications: Warms yang, dispels cold, moves the qi, and resolves fish and meat toxins; treats abdominal distention and pain, indigestion, scanty appetite, vomiting, and low back pain.

Duck

Nature, flavor & channel entering: Sweet and level; enters the lung and kidney channels.

Functions & indications: Moistens dryness and enriches yin, nourishes the stomach and engenders fluids; treats dry cough and vexatious heat and thirst.

Eel

Nature, flavor & channel entering: Sweet and warm; enters the liver, spleen, and kidney channels.

Functions & indications: Supplements vacuity detriment, eliminates wind dampness, strengthens the sinews and bones; treats consumptive damage, wind cold damp impediment, postpartum dribbling urinary block, dysentery with pus and blood, and hemorrhoids.

Eggplant

Nature, flavor & channel entering: Sweet and cool; enters the large intestine, stomach, and spleen channels.

Functions & indications: Clears heat and cools the blood, quickens the blood and transforms stasis; treats hemorrhoidal bleeding, breast abscesses, and swellings and sores.

Fennel

Nature, flavor & channel entering: Acrid and warm; enters the liver, kidney, spleen, and stomach channels.

Functions & indications: Courses the liver, rectifies the qi, and harmonizes the stomach; treats cold mounting pain, flatulence, abdominal distention, indigestion, reduced appetite, vomiting, and qi stagnation menstrual pain.

Fig

Nature, flavor & channel entering: Sweet and level; enters the spleen, stomach, and large intestine channels.

Functions & indications: Fortifies the spleen and harmonizes the stomach, engenders fluids and frees the stool; treats lack of appetite and indigestion, fluid dryness constipation, dry, sore throat and dry cough.

Frog

Nature, flavor & channel entering: Sweet and cool; enters the bladder, intestines, and stomach channels.

Functions & indications: Clears heat and resolves toxins, supplements vacuity, disinhibits water and disperses swelling; treats taxation fever, superficial edema, welling abscess accumulations, water swelling, diaphragmatic occlusion, dysentery, and pediatric heat sores.

Garlic

Nature, flavor & channel entering: Acrid and warm; enters the spleen, stomach, and lung channels.

Functions & indications: Moves stagnant qi, warms the spleen and stomach, disperses concretions and accumulations, resolves toxins, and kills worms; treats food and drink accumulation and stagnation, epigastric chilly pain, water swelling, distention, and fullness, diarrhea, dysentery, malaria-like diseases, whooping cough, welling and flat abscesses, and swelling toxins.

Ginger (dry)
Nature, flavor & channel entering: Acrid and hot; enters the spleen, stomach, and lung channels.

Functions & indications: Warms the center and dispels cold, returns yang and frees the flow of the vessels; treats heart and abdominal chilly pain, vomiting and diarrhea, chilled limbs, a faint pulse, cold rheum panting and coughing, wind cold damp impediment, yang vacuity vomiting and epistaxis, and precipitation of blood.

Ginger (uncooked)
Nature, flavor & channel entering: Acrid and slightly warm; enters the spleen, stomach, and lung channels.

Functions & indications: Resolves the exterior and scatters cold, stops vomiting and transforms phlegm; treats wind cold common cold, vomiting phlegm fluids, and cough with profuse phlegm.

Grape
Nature, flavor & channel entering: Sweet, sour, and level; enters the lung, spleen, and kidney channels.

Functions & indications: Supplements the qi and blood, strengthens the sinews and bones, disinhibits urination; treats qi and blood vacuity weakness, lung vacuity cough, heart palpitations, night sweats, wind damp impediment pain, strangury conditions, and edema.

Grapefruit
Nature, flavor & channel entering: Sweet, sour, and cold; enters the lung, spleen, and stomach channels.

Functions & indications: Rectifies the qi and downbears counterflow, engenders fluids and transforms phlegm; treats dry cough with phlegm, indigestion, burping and belching, mouth watering during pregnancy, and the ill effects of alcohol intoxication.

Grapefruit peel
Nature, flavor & channel entering: Acrid, sweet, bitter, and warm; enters the spleen, kidney, and bladder channels.

Functions & indications: Rectifies the qi and downbears counterflow, eliminates dampness and transforms phlegm; treats nausea and vomiting, abdominal distention and pain, indigestion and diarrhea in children.

Green bean (a.k.a. string bean)
Nature, flavor & channel entering: Sweet and level; enters the spleen and kidney channels.

Functions & indications: Supplements the spleen and kidneys; treats diarrhea, vomiting, wasting thirst, white vaginal discharge, seminal emission, and frequent, numerous urination.

Guava
Nature, flavor & channel entering: Sweet, astringent, and warm; enters the lung, spleen, intestines and stomach channels.

Functions & indications: Supplements the spleen and engenders fluids, secures, astringes, stops diarrhea; treats wasting thirst, pediatric diarrhea, and hoarse throat.

Hazelnut
Nature, flavor & channel entering: Sweet, aromatic, slimy, and level; enters the spleen and stomach channels.

Functions & indications: Fortifies the spleen and opens the stomach, supplements the qi and blood, brightens the eyes; treats qi and blood vacuity weakness, emaciation, malnutrition, chronic diarrhea, and pediatric diarrhea.

Honey

Nature, flavor & channel entering: Sweet, glossy, and level; enters the lung, spleen, and large intestine channels.

Functions & indications: Supplements the center and moistens dryness, relaxes tension and resolves toxins; treats lung dryness cough, intestinal dryness constipation, stomach venter aching and pain, runny nose, mouth sores, and scalding burns (when applied externally).

Job's tears barley

Nature, flavor & channel entering: Sweet, bland, and slightly cold; enters the spleen, lung, and kidney channels.

Functions & indications: Fortifies the spleen and stops diarrhea, disinhibits urination and seeps dampness, clears heat and expels pus, dispels wind dampness, clears and eliminates damp heat; treats various urinary difficulties, edema, leg qi, diarrhea, purulent sores and lung or intestinal abscesses, wind damp impediment, and various damp conditions of the intestines and skin.

Kelp

Nature, flavor & channel entering: Salty and cold; enters the kidney, liver, lung, and stomach channels.

Functions & indications: Softens hardness and transforms phlegm, disinhibits water and drains heat; treats scrofulas, concretions and conglomerations, water swelling, and foot qi.

Kiwi fruit

Nature, flavor & channel entering: Sour, sweet, and cool; enters the spleen and stomach channels.

Functions & indications: Clears heat and engenders fluids, fortifies the spleen and stops diarrhea; treats fever with dry, painful throat, burning heat in the epigastrium with vomiting, jaundice due to damp heat, red, painful urination, indigestion, loss of appetite, and diarrhea due to spleen vacuity.

Kumquat

Nature, flavor & channel entering: Acrid, sweet, slightly sour, and warm; enters the liver, spleen, and stomach channels.

Functions & indications: Rectifies the qi and harmonizes the stomach, dries dampness and transforms phlegm; treats abdominal distention and pain, nausea and indigestion, mounting pain, and cough with thin, clear phlegm.

Lamb

Nature, flavor & channel entering: Sweet and warm; enters the spleen and kidney channels.

Functions & indications: Boosts the qi and supplements vacuity, warms the center and warms below; treats vacuity taxation emaciation and cachexia, low back and knee soreness and weakness, postpartum vacuity chill, abdominal pain, cold mounting, and central vacuity hiccup.

Lemon

Nature, flavor & channel entering: Sour, astringent, and warm; enters the lung, spleen, and stomach channels.

Functions & indications: Transforms phlegm and stops cough, engenders fluids and supplements the spleen; treats vexatious thirst, dry, painful throat, indigestion, and cough with profuse phlegm.

Lettuce

Nature, flavor & channel entering: Bitter, sweet, and cool; enters the stomach and large intestine channels.

Functions & indications: Clears heat, disinhibits urination, and promotes lactation; treats difficult urination, hematuria, and scanty lactation.

Litchi

Nature, flavor & channel entering: Sweet, slightly sour, and warm; enters the liver, spleen, and stomach channels.

Functions & indications: Engenders fluids and boosts the blood, rectifies the qi and stops pain; treats vexatious thirst, qi and blood vacuity weakness, spleen vacuity diarrhea, and stomach pain.

Longan

Nature, flavor & channel entering: Sweet and warm; enters the heart and spleen channels.

Functions & indications: Nourishes the heart and supplements the spleen; treats insomnia, heart palpitations, impaired memory, restlessness, blurred vision, and dizziness due to qi and blood dual vacuity.

Loquat

Nature, flavor & channel entering: Sweet or sweet and sour and cool; enters the lung, spleen, and stomach channels.

Functions & indications: Clears heat, moistens the lungs, stops thirst, and downbears the qi; treats dry, sore throat, vexatious thirst, and dry cough.

Lotus root

Nature, flavor & channel entering: Sweet and cold; enters the heart, spleen, and stomach channels.

Functions & indications: Clears heat, cools the blood, and scatters stasis; treats vexatious thirst due to heat disease, epistaxis, hematemesis, and heat strangury.

Lotus seed

Nature, flavor & channel entering: Sweet, astringent, and level; enters the heart, kidney, and spleen channels.

Functions & indications: Supplements the spleen and stops diarrhea, supplements the kidneys and secures the essence, nourishes the heart and quiets the spirit; treats loss of appetite, chronic diarrhea, premature ejaculation, seminal emission, heart palpitations, insomnia, and restlessness.

Mango

Nature, flavor & channel entering: Sweet, sour, and cool; enters the lung, spleen, and stomach channels.

Functions & indications: Rectifies the qi and downbears counterflow, fortifies the spleen and boosts the stomach; treats cough, panting and wheezing, vomiting, and indigestion.

Marjoram

Nature, flavor & channel entering: Acrid and cool; enters the lung, spleen, and stomach channels.

Functions & indications: Resolves the exterior and clears summerheat, disinhibits urination and opens the stomach; treats summerheat, water swelling, and lack of appetite and bad breath due to food accumulation.

Milk (human)

Nature, flavor & channel entering: Sweet, salty, and level; enters the five viscera and stomach channels.

Functions & indications: Supplements the blood and fills humors, fosters the essence and engenders muscle (*i.e.*, flesh), transforms qi and quiets the spirit, boosts intelligence, grows the sinews and bones, disinhibits the joints, strengthens the stomach and nourishes the spleen, sharpens the hearing and brightens the eyes.

Milk (cow)

Nature, flavor & channel entering: Sweet and level; enters the heart, lung, and stomach channels.

Functions & indications: Supplements vacuity detriment, boosts the lungs and stomach, engenders fluids and moistens the intestines; treats vacuity weakness and taxation detriment, hiccup, diaphragmatic occlusion, wasting thirst, and fluid dryness constipation.

Milk (goat)

Nature, flavor & channel entering: Sweet and warm; enters the lung, kidney, and stomach channels.

Functions & indications: Warms, moistens, and supplements vacuity, supplements the lung and kidney qi, harmonizes the small intestine, boosts the essence qi; treats vacuity taxation emaciation and weakness, wasting thirst, hiccup, burping, and mouth sores.

Millet

Nature, flavor & channel entering: Sweet, salty, and cool; enters the kidney, spleen & stomach channels.

Functions & indications: Harmonizes the stomach and boosts the kidneys, eliminates heat and resolves toxins; treats spleen-stomach vacuity heat, stomach qi counterflow vomiting, wasting thirst, and diarrhea.

Molasses

Nature, flavor & channel entering: Sweet and warm; enters the lung, spleen, and stomach channels.

Functions & indications: Fortifies the spleen and boosts the qi, moistens the lungs and engenders fluids; treats abdominal distention and pain associated with spleen qi vacuity and dry cough with lung yin vacuity.

Mulberry

Nature, flavor & channel entering: Sweet, or sour and sweet, cool; enters the lung, spleen, liver, and kidney channels.

Functions & indications: Supplements vacuity and stops cough, disinhibits urination, disperses swelling, supplements the kidneys and brightens the eyes, nourishes the blood and supplements the liver; treats blurred vision and night blindness due to liver-kidney dual vacuity, dizziness, tinnitus, premature greying of hair, and wasting thirst.

Mung bean

Nature, flavor & channel entering: Sweet and cool; enters the heart and stomach channels.

Functions & indications: Clears heat and resolves toxins, disperses summerheat and disinhibits water; treats summerheat heat, vexatious thirst, water swelling, diarrhea and dysentery, cinnabar toxins, welling abscesses and swellings, and medicinal toxicity.

Mushroom

Nature, flavor & channel entering: Sweet and cool; enters the intestines, stomach, and lung channels.

Functions & indications: Opens the stomach, rectifies the qi, transforms phlegm, quiets the spirit, resolves toxins, out-thrusts rashes, and stops vomiting and diarrhea; treats the latter stages of heat diseases, bodily fatigue and qi weakness, dry mouth with no eating, cough with phlegm, chest and diaphragmatic oppression and fullness, vomiting and diarrhea, and pediatric measles rash which is not easily out-thrust.

Mussel

Nature, flavor & channel entering: Salty and warm; enters the liver and kidney channels.

Functions & indications: Supplements the kidneys and invigorates yang, nourishes the liver and strengthens the sinews, moistens dryness and fills the essence; treats dizziness and vertigo, night sweats, impotence, low back pain, vaginal bleeding, and abnormal vaginal discharge due to liver-kidney dual vacuity.

Mustard green

Nature, flavor & channel entering: Acrid and warm; enters the lung and stomach channel.

Functions & indications: Warms and resolves the exterior, transforms phelgm and scatters cold, rectifies the qi and blood, and warms the center; treats cold phlegm, cough and panting with profuse, white phlegm, and chest oppression.

Nutmeg

Nature, flavor & channel entering: Acrid and warm; enters the large intestine, spleen, and stomach channels.

Functions & indications: Secures the intestines and stops diarrhea, warms the center and moves the qi; treats enduring, hard to treat diarrhea or cockcrow diarrhea due to spleen-kidney vacuity, abdominal distention and pain, and vomiting due to spleen-stomach vacuity.

Oat

Nature, flavor & channel entering: Sweet and level; enters the spleen, stomach, lung, and large intestine channels.

Functions & indications: Fortifies the spleen, boosts the qi, and moistens dryness; treats spontaneous perspiration due to vacuity and fluid dryness of the intestines.

Olive
Nature, flavor & channel entering: Sweet, sour, astringent, and level; enters the lung and stomach channels.

Functions & indications: Astringes and secures, engenders fluids and moistens the lungs; treats dry, sore throat, dry cough, hemoptysis, enduring diarrhea and dysentery, and hangover due to alcohol.

Onion
Nature, flavor & channel entering: Acrid and warm; enters the lung, spleen, liver, and large intestine channels.

Functions & indications: Warms the internal and scatters cold, resolves the exterior and dispels wind, moves the qi and quickens the blood; treats wind cold common cold, diarrhea, and worms.

Orange
Nature, flavor & channel entering: Sweet, sour, and cool; enters the lung and stomach channels.

Functions & indications: Opens the stomach and rectifies the qi, stops thirst and moistens the lungs; treats chest and diaphragmatic bound qi, counterflow vomiting and scanty eating, stomach yin insufficiency, dry thirst within the mouth, lung heat cough, and excessive drinking of alcohol.

Orange peel
Nature, flavor & channel entering: Sour, bitter, aromatic, and warm; enters the lung, spleen, and stomach channels.

Functions & indications: Rectifies the qi and moves the spleen, harmonizes the center and loosens the diaphragm, dries dampness and transforms phlegm; treats indigestion, abdominal distention and pain, hiccup, burping and belching, nausea and vomiting, phlegm damp cough, chest oppression, profuse phlegm, damp turbidity obstructing the center, and lack of appetite.

Oyster
Nature, flavor & channel entering: Salty, sweet, and level; enters the liver and kidney channels.

Functions & indications: Supplements the liver and kidneys; treats insomnia, restlessness, and agitation.

Papaya
Nature, flavor & channel entering: Sweet, cold, and level; enters the spleen and stomach channels.

Functions & indications: Fortifies the spleen and stomach, clears summerheat and resolves thirst; treats fever with vexatious thirst, persistent cough, scanty lactation, and indigestion.

Pea
Nature, flavor & channel entering: Sweet and level; enters the heart, spleen, stomach, and large intestine channels.

Functions & indications: Fortifies the spleen and disinhibits urination, moistens the intestines and frees the flow of the stool; treats indigestion due to spleen-stomach vacuity weakness, edema, and fluid dryness constipation.

Peach
Nature, flavor & channel entering: Sweet, sour, and warm; enters the intestine and stomach channels.

Functions & indications: Engenders fluids and moistens the intestines, quickens the blood and disperses accumulations.

Peanut
Nature, flavor & channel entering: Sweet and level; enters the spleen and lung channels.

Functions & indications: Moistens the lungs, harmonizes the

stomach, and stops bleeding; treats dry cough, nausea, foot qi, and scanty lactation.

Pear

Nature, flavor & channel entering: Sweet, slightly sour, and cool; enters the lung and stomach channels.

Functions & indications: Engenders fluids and moistens dryness, clears heat and transforms phlegm; treats heat disease damaging fluids, vexatious thirst, wasting thirst, heat cough, phlegm heat, fright mania, diaphragmatic occlusion, and constipation.

Peppermint

Nature, flavor & channel entering: Acrid and cool; enters the lung and liver channels.

Functions & indications: Clears heat and resolves the exterior, clears the head and eyes and disinhibits the throat, out-thrusts rashes, courses the liver and rectifies the qi; treats wind heat common cold with fever, headache, cough, sore throat, red eyes, the early stage of measles, abdominal and rib-side distention and pain, irritability, and premenstrual breast and abdominal distention and pain.

Persimmon

Nature, flavor & channel entering: Sweet, astringent, and cold; enters the lung, spleen, and stomach channels.

Functions & indications: Moistens the lungs, engenders fluids, and fortifies the spleen; treats epigastric heat and pain, coughing and wheezing, diarrhea and dysentery, bleeding hemorrhoids, high blood pressure, sores in the mouth, dry, painful throat, and incessant hiccups.

Pineapple
Nature, flavor & channel entering: Sweet, slightly astringent, and level; enters the spleen and stomach channels.

Functions & indications: Supplements the spleen, engenders fluids, and dispels wind dampness; treats indigestion, vomiting, abdominal distention, low blood pressure, lack of strength in the hands and feet, vacuity fever with thirst, and difficulty urinating.

Pine nut
Nature, flavor & channel entering: Sweet and warm; enters the liver, lung, and large intestine channels.

Functions & indications: Nourishes fluids, extinguishes wind, and moistens the lungs and large intestine; treats wind impediment, dizziness, dry cough, hematemesis, and constipation.

Plum
Nature, flavor & channel entering: Bitter, sour, astringent, and cool; enters the spleen, stomach, and bladder channels.

Functions & indications: Clears heat, disinhibits urination, and promotes digestion; treats indigestion, bleeding gums, gingivitis, chronic inflammation of the throat, and sores on the tongue and in the mouth.

Pomegranate
Nature, flavor & channel entering: Sweet, sour, astringent, and cool; enters the lung, spleen, and stomach channels.

Functions & indications: Clears heat, moistens the lungs, and stops cough; treats dry, sore throat, hoarse voice, enduring cough, diarrhea and dysentery, and damp heat skin lesions.

Pomelo
Nature, flavor & channel entering: Sweet, sour, and cool; enters the lung, spleen, and stomach channels.

Functions & indications: Fortifies the spleen, transforms phlegm, stops cough, and resolves alcohol toxins; treats cough with profuse phlegm, nausea, vomiting, and indigestion, hangover from alcohol, wind damp impediment, and swelling due to falls and knocks.

Pork

Nature, flavor & channel entering: Sweet, salty, and level; enters the spleen, stomach, and kidney channels.

Functions & indications: Supplements the kidneys and nourishes the blood, enriches yin and moistens dryness; treats heat disease damaging fluids, wasting thirst, kidney vacuity constitutional weakness, postpartum blood vacuity, dry cough, and fluid dryness constipation.

Potato

Nature, flavor & channel entering: Sweet and level or slightly cold; enters the spleen and stomach channels.

Functions & indications: Supplements the spleen and boosts the qi (when eaten cooked), clears heat and resolves toxins (when the juice is drunk or applied externally); treats acute hepatitis, breast abscesses, laryngitis, tonsillitis, mumps, and stomach and duodenal ulcers.

Pumpkin (& other winter squash)

Nature, flavor & channel entering: Sweet and warm; enters the spleen and stomach channels.

Functions & indications: Supplements the center and boosts the qi, disperses inflammation and stops pain, resolves toxins and kills worms.

Pumpkin seed

Nature, flavor & channel entering: Sweet and warm; enters the spleen, stomach and large intestine channels.

Functions & indications: Kills worms, moistens the intestines and frees the flow of the stool; treats parasites, bleeding hemorrhoids, and scanty lactation.

Purslane

Nature, flavor & channel entering: Sour and cold; enters the large intestine, liver, and spleen channels.

Functions & indications: Clears heat and resolves toxins, scatters the blood and disperses swelling; treats heat dysentery with pus and blood, heat strangury, bloody strangury, abnormal vaginal discharge, and welling abscesses and swellings, malign sores, cinnabar toxins, and scrofulas (when applied externally).

Radish

Nature, flavor & channel entering: Acrid, sweet, and cool; enters the lung and stomach channels.

Functions & indications: Disperses accumulations and stagnation, transforms phlegm and clears heat, descends the qi, broadens the center, and resolves toxins; treats food accumulation, distention and fullness, phlegm cough, hematemesis, epistaxis, wasting thirst, dysentery, and migraine headache.

Raspberry

Nature, flavor & channel entering: Sour, sweet, and warm; enters the liver and kidney channels.

Functions & indications: Nourishes the liver and enriches the kidneys, secures and astringes; treats liver-kidney yin vacuity, seminal emission, and frequent, numerous urination.

Red date

Nature, flavor & channel entering: Sweet and level; enters the spleen and stomach channels.

Functions & indications: Supplements the spleen and boosts the qi, nourishes the blood and quiets the spirit; treats qi and blood vacuity weakness with fatigue, shortness of breath, scanty appetite, and loose stools, and irritability and restlessness due to visceral agitation.

Rice

Nature, flavor & channel entering: Sweet and level; enters the spleen & stomach channels.

Functions & indications: Supplements the center and boosts the qi, fortifies the spleen and harmonizes the stomach; eliminates vexatious thirst, stops diarrhea and dysentery.

Rice (glutinous)

Nature, flavor & channel entering: Sweet and warm; enters the lung, spleen, and stomach channels.

Functions & indications: Supplements the lungs and fortifies the spleen; stops diarrhea and spontaneous perspiration.

Rosemary

Nature, flavor & channel entering: Acrid and warm; enters the lung and stomach channels.

Functions & indications: Resolves the exterior and scatters cold, moves the qi and opens the stomach; treats wind cold common cold, headache, abdominal pain, indigestion, and menstrual pain.

Russian olive

Nature, flavor & channel entering: Sweet or sour and sweet, and level; enters the lung, liver, spleen, kidney, and stomach channels.

Functions & indications: Supplements the spleen and stomach, nourishes the liver and moistens the lungs; treats indigestion, abdominal distention and pain, pediatric diarrhea, seminal emission, profuse menstruation, blurred vision, impaired memory, insomnia, cough with scanty or no phlegm, and menopausal dryness complaints.

Saffron

Nature, flavor & channel entering: Sweet and level or warm; enters the heart and liver channels.

Functions & indications: Quickens the blood, transforms stasis, and stops pain; treats blood stasis patterns of blocked menstruation (*i.e.*, amenorrhea), painful menstruation, postpartum dizziness, concretions and conglomerations, heart and chest pain, and injuries due to falls and knocks.

Salt

Nature, flavor & channel entering: Salty and cold; enters the stomach, kidney, large intestine, and small intestine channels.

Functions & indications: Induces vomiting and disperses phlegm (when used as an emetic), cools the blood and clears fire, resolves toxins; treats food collected in the upper venter, heart and abdominal distention and pain, phlegm accumulated in the chest, non-free flow of urination and defecation, bleeding gums, sore throat, toothache, eye screen, sores, and toxins due to snake and insect bite.

Scallion

Nature, flavor & channel entering: Acrid and warm; enters the lung and stomach channels.

Functions & indications: Emits the exterior, frees the flow of yang, and resolves toxins; treats cold damage with fever and chills and headache, yin cold abdominal pain, worm accumulation obstructing internally, non-free flow of urination and defecation, dysentery, and welling abscesses and swellings (when applied externally).

Sesame (black or yellow)
Nature, flavor & channel entering: Sweet and level; enters the liver and kidney channels.

Functions & indications: Supplements the liver and kidneys, moistens the five viscera; treats liver-kidney insufficiency, vacuity wind dizziness and vertigo, wind impediment, paralysis, large intestine dry binding, premature whitening of the hair, and scanty lactation in women.

Shark
Nature, flavor & channel entering: Sweet, salty, and level; enters the five viscera and stomach channels.

Functions & indications: Boosts the qi, supplements vacuity, and opens the stomach.

Shepherd's purse
Nature, flavor & channel entering: Sweet and level; enters the liver, heart, lung, and spleen channels.

Functions & indications: Harmonizes the spleen, disinhibits water, stops bleeding, and brightens the eyes; treats dysentery, water swelling, strangury conditions, hematemesis, epistaxis, hemafecia, profuse menstruation, flooding and leaking, and red, swollen, painful eyes.

Shrimp
Nature, flavor & channel entering: Sweet and warm; enters the liver and kidney channels.

Functions & indications: Nourishes the liver and invigorates the kidneys; treats impotence and scanty lactation.

Sichuan pepper
Nature, flavor & channel entering: Acrid, hot, and slightly toxic; enters the kidney, spleen, and stomach channels.

Functions & indications: Warms the center and scatters cold, kills worms and stops pain; treats chilly pain in the abdomen, vomiting and diarrhea, and abdominal pain due to worms.

Sorghum
Nature, flavor & channel entering: Sweet and warm; enters the spleen and stomach channels.

Functions & indications: Warms the center and fortifies the spleen, seeps dampness and stops dysentery; treats spleen vacuity with damp encumbrance, indigestion, damp heat precipitating dysentery, and inhibited urination.

Soybean (black)
Nature, flavor & channel entering: Sweet and level; enters the spleen and large intestine channels.

Functions & indications: Quickens the blood and disinhibits water, dispels wind and resolves toxins; treats water swelling, distention and fullness, wind toxins, foot qi, jaundice, edema, wind impediment, sinew contraction, postpartum wind tetany, welling abscesses and swellings, and sore toxins.

Soybean (yellow)
Nature, flavor & channel entering: Sweet and level; enters the spleen and large intestine channels.

Functions & indications: Fortifies the spleen and loosens the intestines, moistens dryness and disperses water; treats *gan* accumulation diarrhea and dysentery, abdominal distention, emaciation, toxemia during pregnancy, sores and welling abscesses, swelling toxins, bleeding due to external injury.

Soybean sprout

Nature, flavor & channel entering: Sweet and cool; enters the spleen, stomach, and large intestine channels.

Functions & indications: Clears heat and disinhibits urination, harmonizes the stomach and disperses accumulations; treats food stagnation, heat in the stomach, edema, and damp heat impediment.

Soy sauce

Nature, flavor & channel entering: Salty and cold; enters the stomach, spleen, and kidney channels.

Functions & indications: Eliminates heat and resolves toxins; treats bee and wasp sting, scalds and burns (when applied externally), and vexation and fullness in heat diseases.

Spearmint

Nature, flavor & channel entering: Acrid and warm; enters the lung, liver, and stomach channels.

Functions & indications: Resolves the exterior and scatters cold, moves the qi and stops pain; treats indigestion, abdominal pain, wind cold common cold, headache, and menstrual pain.

Spinach

Nature, flavor & channel entering: Sweet and cool; enters the large intestine and stomach channels.

Functions & indications: Nourishes the blood and stops bleeding, astringes yin and moistens dryness; treats epistaxis, hemafecia, frequent drinking due to wasting thirst, and constipation.

Squash (summer, including cucumber)
Nature, flavor & channel entering: Sweet and cold; enters the spleen, stomach, and large intestine channels.

Functions & indications: Clears heat and disinhibits water, resolves toxins and disperses inflammation, stops thirst and quiets agitation; treats difficulty urinating, edema, summerheat, irritability, and oral thirst.

Squid
Nature, flavor & channel entering: Salty, sweet, and level; enters the liver and kidney channels.

Functions & indications: Nourishes the liver and enriches the kidneys; treats blood vacuity, vaginal bleeding and vaginal discharge, and blocked menstruation (*i.e.*, amenorrhea).

Strawberry
Nature, flavor & channel entering: Sweet, sour, and cool; enters the lung, spleen, liver, kidney, and stomach channels.

Functions & indications: Moistens the lungs and engenders fluids, supplements and nourishes the liver and kidneys, astringes and secures; treats dry cough with no or scanty phlegm, sore, swollen throat, lack of appetite and indigestion, frequent, numerous urination, hangover from alcohol, dizziness, and vacuity weakness after enduring disease.

Sugar (brown)
Nature, flavor & channel entering: Sweet and warm; enters the liver, spleen, and stomach channels.

Functions & indications: Supplements the spleen and boosts the qi, quickens the blood and transforms stasis; treats abdominal pain, dysentery, and lower abdominal pain due to non insufficient or non-precipitation of the lochia after childbirth.

Sugar (white)
Nature, flavor & channel entering: Sweet and level; enters the lung and spleen channels.

Functions & indications: Supplements the center and boosts the qi, harmonizes the center and moistens the lungs; treats lung dryness, lung vacuity, wind cold, taxation and fatigue, coughing and panting, pediatric malaria-like disease, mouth sores, and wind fire toothache.

Sunflower seed
Nature, flavor & channel entering: Sweet and level; channel entry not yet established

Functions & indications: Supplements the spleen and moistens the intestines, stops dysentery and disperses welling abscesses; treats intestinal dryness constipation, dysentery with pus and blood, and welling abscesses and swellings that have not yet broken.

Sweet potato
Nature, flavor & channel entering: Sweet and level or cool; enters the spleen and stomach channels.

Functions & indications: Fortifies the spleen and supplements the qi, enriches the kidneys and engenders fluids; treats diarrhea, constipation, wasting thirst, kidney yin vacuity, and premature ejaculation.

Tea (green)
Nature, flavor & channel entering: Bitter, sweet, and cool; enters the heart, lung, and stomach channels.

Functions & indications: Clears the head and eyes, eliminates vexatious thirst, transforms phlegm, disperses food, disinhibits urination, and resolves toxins; treats headache, dizziness, excessive sleeping, lack of clarity of thinking, heart vexation, oral thirst, food accumulation, phlegm stagnation, and dysentery.

Thyme

Nature, flavor & channel entering: Acrid and warm; enters the lung and stomach channels.

Functions & indications: Resolves the exterior and dispels cold, moves the qi and opens the stomach, downbears counterflow and stops cough; treats wind cold common cold with headache, cough, bodily aches and pains, and sore throat, whooping cough, nausea, vomiting, indigestion, and abdominal distention.

Tofu

Nature, flavor & channel entering: Sweet and cool; enters the spleen, stomach, and large intestine channels.

Functions & indications: Boosts the qi and harmonizes the center, engenders fluids and moistens dryness, clears heat and resolves toxins; treats red eyes, wasting thirst, and recurrent dysentery.

Tomato

Nature, flavor & channel entering: Sweet, sour, and slightly cold; enters the stomach channel.

Functions & indications: Clears heat and levels the liver, moistens dryness and stops thirst, opens the stomach and disperses accumulations, quickens the blood and transforms stasis; treats mouth sores, wasting thirst, red eyes, dizziness, and food damage indigestion.

Turmeric

Nature, flavor & channel entering: Acrid, bitter, and warm; enters the spleen, stomach, and liver channels.

Functions & indications: Quickens the blood and frees the flow of menstruation, moves the qi and stops pain, dispels wind dampness; treats blocked menstruation (*i.e.*,amenorrhea), painful menstruation, pain and swelling due to traumatic injury, epigastric and abdominal pain, and wind damp painful impediment.

Turnip

Nature, flavor & channel entering: Acrid, bitter, and cool; enters the spleen, stomach, and lung channels.

Functions & indications: Clears heat and eliminates dampness, disperses food accumulation and stagnation, transforms phlegm and stops cough, resolves toxins; treats breast abscesses, phlegm heat cough, and food stagnation indigestion complicated by heat.

Umeboshi

Nature, flavor & channel entering: Sour and warm; enters the large intestine, liver, lung, and spleen channels.

Functions & indications: Secures the lung qi and stops cough, secures the intestines and stops diarrhea, engenders fluids and resolves thirst, kills worms and stops bleeding; treats lung qi vacuity cough, enduring diarrhea and dysentery, thirst, including wasting thirst, abdominal pain and vomiting from worms and intestinal dysbiosis, and hemafecia and uterine bleeding due to qi vacuity.

Venison

Nature, flavor & channel entering: Sweet and warm; enters the liver and kidney channels.

Functions & indications: Nourishes the liver and invigorates the kidneys, strengthens the sinews and bones; treats low back and knee soreness and weakness, premature ejaculation, impotence, and sterility.

Vinegar

Nature, flavor & channel entering: Sour, bitter, and warm; enters the liver and stomach channels.

Functions & indications: Scatters stasis, stops bleeding, resolves toxins, and kills worms; treats postpartum blood dizziness, string like concretions and conglomerations, jaundice, yellow sweating, hematemesis, epistaxis, hemafecia, vaginal itching, and welling and flat abscesses, sores and swellings.

Walnut
Nature, flavor & channel entering: Sweet and warm; enters the kidney and lung channels.

Functions & indications: Supplements the kidneys and secures the essence, warms the lungs and stabilizes panting, moistens the intestines and frees the flow of the stool; treats kidney vacuity wheezing and coughing, low back pain and lower leg weakness, impotence, seminal emission, frequent, numerous urination, stone strangury, and large intestine dryness and binding.

Water chestnut
Nature, flavor & channel entering: Sweet, bland, and cool; enters the lung, spleen, stomach, large intestine, and bladder channels.

Functions & indications: Clears heat and transforms phlegm, engenders fluids and disinhibits urination, lowers blood pressure; treats lung heat with sticky, difficult to expectorate phlegm, dry, painful throat, fever with thirst, wasting thirst, red, scanty, painful urination, jaundice, red, painful eyes, measles, dysentery with blood in the stools, bleeding hemorrhoids, and hypertension.

Watercress
Nature, flavor & channel entering: Acrid, bitter, and cool; enters the lung, stomach, and bladder channels.

Functions & indications: Clears heat and stops thirst, moistens the lungs and disinhibits urination; treats vexatious thirst, restlessness and irritability, dry, sore throat, and cough with yellow phlegm.

Watermelon

Nature, flavor & channel entering: Sweet and cold; enters the heart, stomach, and bladder channels.

Functions & indications: Clears heat and resolves summerheat, eliminates vexation and stops thirst, disinhibits urination; treats summerheat heat, vexatious thirst, heat exuberance damaging fluids, inhibition of urination, oral sores, and throat impediment.

Wheat

Nature, flavor & channel entering: Sweet and cool; enters the heart, spleen and kidney channels.

Functions & indications: Nourishes the heart and boosts the kidneys, eliminates heat and stops thirst; treats visceral agitation, vexatious heat, wasting thirst, diarrhea and dysentery, welling abscesses and swellings, and bleeding due to external injury.

White fungus

Nature, flavor & channel entering: Sweet, bland, glossy, and level; enters the lung and stomach channels.

Functions & indications: Enriches yin, moistens the lungs, and engenders fluids; treats insomnia, dry cough, and yin vacuity-fluid dryness conditions in general.

Yogurt

Nature, flavor & channel entering: Sweet, sour, and warm; enters the lung, liver, stomach, and large intestine channels.

Functions & indications: Moistens the lungs and large intestine, eliminates vexation and resolves thirst; treats dry cough and fluid dryness constipation.

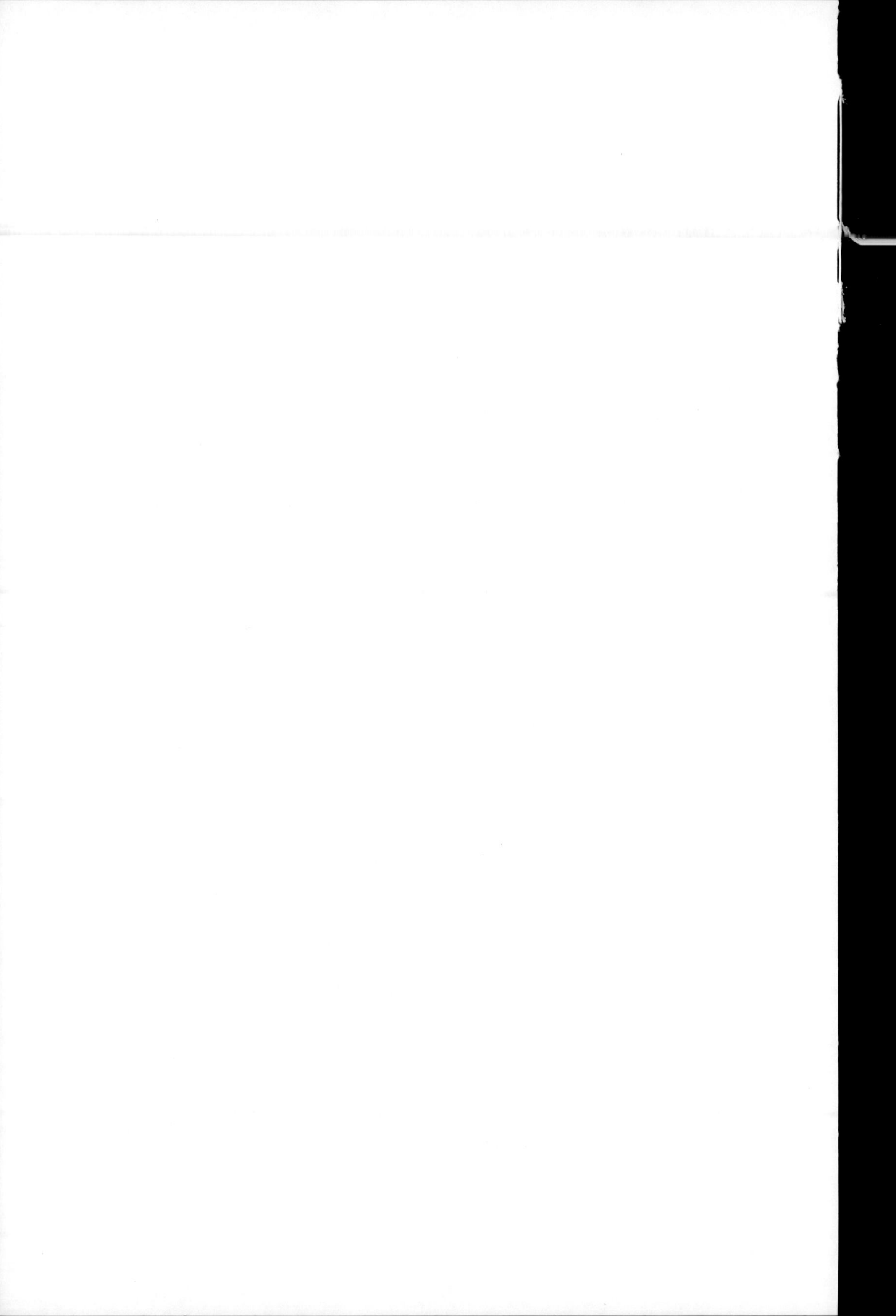

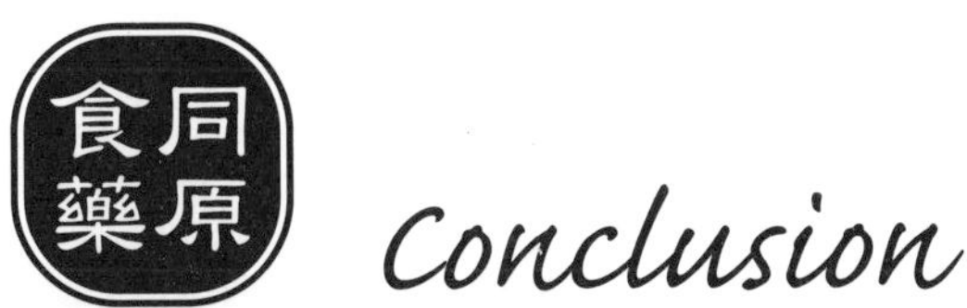

Conclusion

While preparing this small book on Chinese dietary therapy for laypersons, I have coincidentally come across two things which I think support and underscore the importance of this approach. The first is a scientific study comparing the eating habits of 6,500 rural Chinese and their health with Western eating habits and Westerners' health. This study was undertaken jointly by Oxford University in England, the Chinese Academy for Preventive Medicine in Beijing, and Cornell University in the United States. It was called the Cornell-China-Oxford Project on Nutrition, Health and Environment and is still the largest study of a nation's eating habits of this kind ever undertaken.

For two years, the subjects, aged 34-64, were interviewed about their eating and other health habits, such as drinking alcohol and smoking tobacco. Blood samples were taken to measure their cholesterol and other such things, dietary records were obtained, and foods consumed were weighed and measured. Ninety percent of the Chinese selected for this study were provincials who ate locally raised foods and stuck to a traditional diet. Among the important findings were the facts that:

1. Rural Chinese consume many more vegetables, grains, and fruits than either Americans or Britons.

2. The daily fiber intake of the average rural Chinese is three times higher than the average American.

3. The average rural Chinese derives anywhere from 6-24% of their daily calories from fat compared to 39% for the average American and 45% for the average Briton.

4. In most of the counties included in this study, people ate meat only once per week. In counties where meat was eaten more regularly, rates of cardiovascular disease were also higher.

5. The Chinese in this study ate more total calories daily per pound of body weight than did their American counterparts but there was little obesity, certainly far less than in the U.S.A.

6. The average rural Chinese blood cholesterol level was only 127 milligrams per deciliter compared to 212 milligrams in the U.S.

7. The rates for chronic degenerative diseases are much higher in the U.S. than in China. However, in those areas of China where the intake of animal-based foods is higher, so is the rates for these kinds of diseases.

I believe this study supports the fact that the Chinese do have a special insight into diet and the maintenance of health. Based on the outcomes of this study, the Chinese government is currently taking active steps to keep this traditional diet from giving way to the high fat diet of the West.

The second piece of interesting evidence supporting the wisdom of the Chinese medical approach to healthy eating was recently published in Newsweek (May 27, 1991). The cover article of this issue was devoted to new attitudes about diet and health in the United States. According to that article, the USDA has created what it calls "the Eating Right Pyramid." This is a graphic showing, in its preparers' opinion, the most healthy proportions of foods in one's daily diet. This pyramid makes grains and complex carbohydrates the foundation of the diet. Next comes vegetables and fruits. Then comes dairy products and other animal proteins, and last, under the heading "Use Sparingly," comes fats oils, and sweets.

This is very similar to the diet that Chinese medicine also suggests is the healthiest for most humans living in temperate climates. The only change I would make in this scheme is that I would emphasize more vegetables, since, as a clinician, I know that even those Westerners trying to eat a healthy diet tend to eat too many grain products and too few vegetables. The same article quotes Bonnie Liebman, a nutritionist at the Center for Science in the Public Interest, as saying: "for years, the National Academy of Sciences and the National Cancer Institute have been telling Americans to eat more vegetables." Says CSPI's Liebman, "Most of the meal should be grains, vegetables, and beans, and meats should be used as a condiment." Unfortunately but all too typically, then Secretary of Agriculture, Edward R. Madigan, suspended the publication of this chart presumably due to special interest pressure from the meat and dairy industries.

For sure, some "truths" are culturally limited. Certain mores and behavior may work in one culture or country but not in others. However, I have practiced Chinese medicine in Asia, America, and Europe, and I believe that Chinese medicine is a system of thought about human physiology which is so universally valid that its logic can be applied to any person within any culture in the world. Chinese internal medicine is not simply a collection of medicinals which happen to have originated in China, nor is Chinese dietary therapy limited to wontons and egg drop soup. The fundamental insights of Chinese dietary theory can be applied to any national or regional cuisine since all foods in everyone's stomachs must be turned into 100F soup.

Although more and more, Western science supports the diet rural Chinese have been eating for millennia, the facts of Western science are not something immediately experienced on a human level. Cholesterol, enzymes, proteins, etc. are so removed from everyday experience, that people are prone to unconsciously dismiss them even if, theoretically, they know about them. For most people, these facts exist only as vague abstractions. Chinese medicine, on the other hand, has crafted its theories from metaphors taken from everyday reality. This is based on the perception that whatever goes on within the body is not something apart or fundamentally different from what goes on in the world at large.

Chinese medicine is based on the concept that the human organism is a microcosm of the larger, external macrocosm. As a holographic part of this macrocosm, one can apply the same everyday metaphors one uses to understand the world at large to their own insides. Therefore, the analogies between digestion and a pot on a stove, to a car engine, to a still, and to Economics 101 are both accurate and empowering if seemingly simplistic. My experience as a clinician is that such explanations are able to influence the behavior of patients that more abstract explanations often cannot. It is my experience that when we really understand something as being immediately and undeniably true, we tend to act upon that belief.

Chinese dietary therapy gives us a set of explanations from our normal, everyday world. These explanations make sense and, more than that, when they are put into action, they work. As a human being and as a doctor, there are many things which I say I believe but really do not know for sure. But, when it comes to diet, I do know for sure that the wisdom of Chinese dietary therapy does work. I also know that diet is such an important part of our daily life that, unless one's diet is well adjusted, no amount of herbs, acupuncture, or other medicines or treatments can achieve a complete and lasting cure. Therefore, whether for prevention or remedial treatment, proper diet is of the utmost importance, and dietary wisdom is something that everyone needs to know. Chinese medicine has that wisdom and I am offering it to you. Good luck and bon appétit.

食同藥原 Index

C

D

E

F

M

Q

R

S

T

Y

Z

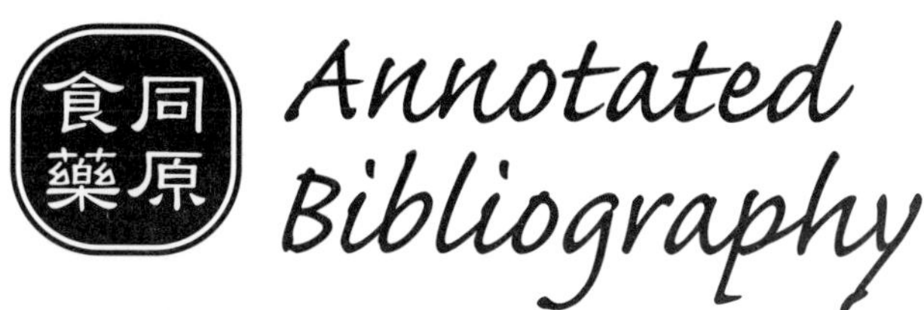

Annotated Bibliography

English Sources

Butt, Gary & Bloomfield, Frena, *Harmony Rules: The Chinese Way of Health Through Food,* Samuel Weiser Inc., York Beach, ME, 1987. This is a layperson's guide to Chinese dietary therapy.

Cai, Jingfeng, *Eating Your Way to Health: Dietotherapy in Traditional Chinese Medicine,* Foreign Languages Press, Beijing, 1988. This book is another layperson's guide to Chinese dietary therapy.

Dai, Yin-fang & Liu, Cheng-jun, *Fruit as Medicine,* trans. by Ron Edwards & Gong Zhi-mei, The Rams Skull Press, Kuranda, Australia, 1987. This book deals with the Chinese medical descriptions and uses of edible fruits.

Flaws, Bob, *The Book of Jook: Chinese Medicinal Porridges, A Healthy Alternative to the Typical Western Breakfast,* Blue Poppy Press, Boulder, CO, 1995. This book discusses the role of porridges in a healthy diet and gives numerous recipes for porridges to treat a wide variety of conditions.

Flaws, Bob, *Chinese Medicinal Wines & Elixirs,* Blue Poppy Press, Boulder, CO, 1994. This book gives scores of recipes for making simple herbal liqueurs and cordials to treat disease and promote health and longevity.

Flaws, Bob, *Food, Phlegm, & Pediatric Disease,* Blue Poppy Press, Boulder, CO, 1990. This pamphlet discusses the pivotal role of diet and feeding in the health of newborns and infants.

Flaws, Bob, *Imperial Secrets of Health & Longevity,* Blue Poppy Press, Boulder, CO, 1994. This book contains a wealth of information on Chinese longevity techniques, including Chinese dietary therapy, written in the same easy-to-understand style as this current book.

Flaws, Bob & Wolfe, Honora Lee, *Prince Wen Hui's Cook: Chinese Dietary Therapy,* Paradigm Publications, Brookline, MA, 1983. This book was an earlier version of a Chinese dietary therapy book for lay readers.

Kaptchuk, Ted, *The Web That Has No Weaver,* Congden & Weed, New York, 1984. This book is still the best layperson's introduction to Chinese medicine available in English.

Leung, Albert Y., *Chinese Herbal Remedies,* Universe Books, New York, 1984. This book contains a lot of interesting information on common foods and herbs and is written with the lay reader in mind.

Liu, Zhengcai, *The Mystery of Longevity,* Foreign Languages Press, Beijing, 1990. This book is an overview of Chinese health and longevity practices and includes a number of self-help treatments for various common diseases.

Lu, Henry C., *Chinese System of Food Cures: Prevention & Remedies,*

Sterling Publishing Co., New York, 1986. This is another layperson's guide to Chinese dietary therapy.

Lu, Henry C., *Legendary Chinese Healing Herbs,* Sterling Publishing Co., New York, 1991. This book is a collection of stories about common Chinese herbs and foods (mostly about how they got their names) written for the lay reader.

Ni, Maoshing & McNease, Cathy, *The Tao of Nutrition,* Shrine of the Eternal Breath of the Tao, Malibu, CA, 1987. This is another layperson's guide to Chinese dietary therapy.

Zhang En-qin, *A Practical English-Chinese Library of Traditional Chinese Medicine: Chinese Medicated Diet,* ed. Shanghai College of Traditional Chinese Medicine Publishing House, Shanghai, 1990. This book covers all the basics of Chinese dietary therapy and includes dietary treatments for many common conditions.

Zong, Xiao-fan & Liscum, Gary, *Chinese Medicinal Teas: Simple, Proven, Folk Formulas for Common Diseases & Promoting Health,* Blue Poppy Press, Boulder, CO, 1996. This book discusses simple herbal teas one can add to one's daily diet to treat disease or promote health and long life.

Chinese Sources

Hu, Hai-tian et al., *Yin Shi Liao Fa* (Drinking & Eating Treatment Methods), Guangdong Science & Technology Press, Guangzhou, 1987

Jiang, Qing-yun, *Shi Zhi Ben Cao* (A Food Treatment Materia Medica), Beijing, 1990

Li Guo-qing et al., *Pian Fang Da Quan* (A Great Collection of Folk Formulas), Beijing Science & Technology Press, Beijing, 1987

Yang, Fei et al., *Da Zhong Yao Shan* (Medicinal Meals of the Masses), Sichuan Science & Technology Press, Chengdu, 1985

Ye, Ku-quan, *Shi Wu Zhong Yao Yu Pian Fang* (Food Stuffs, Chinese Medicinals & Folk Formulas), Jiangsu Science & Technology Press, Nanjing, 1980

OTHER BOOKS ON CHINESE MEDICINE AVAILABLE FROM:

BLUE POPPY PRESS

5441 Western, Suite 2, Boulder, CO 80301
For ordering 1-800-487-9296 PH. 303\447-8372 FAX 303\245-8362
Email: info@bluepoppy.com Website: www.bluepoppy.com

A NEW AMERICAN ACUPUNTURE
By Mark Seem
ISBN 0-936185-44-9

ACUPOINT POCKET REFERENCE
by Bob Flaws
ISBN 0-936185-93-7

ACUPUNCTURE AND MOXIBUSTION FORMULAS & TREATMENTS
by Cheng Dan-an, trans. by Wu Ming
ISBN 0-936185-68-6

ACUPUNCTURE PHYSICAL MEDICINE: An Acupuncture Touchpoint Approach to the Treatment of Chronic Pain, Fatigue, and Stress Disorders
by Mark Seem
ISBN 1-891845-13-6

AGING & BLOOD STASIS: A New Approach to TCM Geriatrics
by Yan De-xin
ISBN 0-936185-63-5

BETTER BREAST HEALTH NATURALLY with CHINESE MEDICINE
by Honora Lee Wolfe & Bob Flaws
ISBN 0-936185-90-2

THE BOOK OF JOOK: Chinese Medicinal Porridges
by Bob Flaws
ISBN 0-936185-60-0

CHANNEL DIVERGENCES Deeper Pathways of the Web
by Miki Shima and Charles Chase
ISBN 1-891845-15-2

CHINESE MEDICAL PALMISTRY: Your Health in Your Hand
by Zong Xiao-fan & Gary Liscum
ISBN 0-936185-64-3

CHINESE MEDICAL PSYCHIATRY A Textbook and Clinical Manual
by Bob Flaws and James Lake, MD
ISBN 1-845891-17-9

CHINESE MEDICINAL TEAS: Simple, Proven, Folk Formulas for Common Diseases & Promoting Health
by Zong Xiao-fan & Gary Liscum
ISBN 0-936185-76-7

CHINESE MEDICINAL WINES & ELIXIRS
by Bob Flaws
ISBN 0-936185-58-9

CHINESE PEDIATRIC MASSAGE THERAPY: A Parent's & Practitioner's Guide to the Prevention & Treatment of Childhood Illness
by Fan Ya-li
ISBN 0-936185-54-6

CHINESE SELF-MASSAGE THERAPY: The Easy Way to Health
by Fan Ya-li
ISBN 0-936185-74-0

CURING ARTHRITIS NATURALLY WITH CHINESE MEDICINE
by Douglas Frank & Bob Flaws
ISBN 0-936185-87-2

CURING DEPRESSION NATURALLY WITH CHINESE MEDICINE
by Rosa Schnyer & Bob Flaws
ISBN 0-936185-94-5

CURING FIBROMYALGIA NATURALLY WITH CHINESE MEDICINE
by Bob Flaws
ISBN 1-891845-08-9

CURING HAY FEVER NATURALLY WITH CHINESE MEDICINE
by Bob Flaws
ISBN 0-936185-91-0

CURING HEADACHES NATURALLY WITH CHINESE MEDICINE
by Bob Flaws
ISBN 0-936185-95-3-X

CURING IBS NATURALLY WITH CHINESE MEDICINE
by Jane Bean Oberski
ISBN 1-891845-11-X

CURING INSOMNIA NATURALLY WITH CHINESE MEDICINE
by Bob Flaws
ISBN 0-936185-85-6

CURING PMS NATURALLY WITH CHINESE MEDICINE
by Bob Flaws
ISBN 0-936185-85-6

A STUDY OF DAOIST ACUPUNCTURE & MOXIBUSTION
by Liu Zheng-cai
ISBN 1-891845-08-X

THE DIVINE FARMER'S MATERIA MEDICA A Translation of the Shen Nong Ben Cao
translation by Yang Shouz-zhong
ISBN 0-936185-96-1

THE DIVINELY RESPONDING CLASSIC: A Translation of the Shen Ying Jing from Zhen Jiu Da Cheng
trans. by Yang Shou-zhong & Liu Feng-ting
ISBN 0-936185-55-4

DUI YAO: THE ART OF COMBINING CHINESE HERBAL MEDICINALS
by Philippe Sionneau
ISBN 0-936185-81-3

ENDOMETRIOSIS, INFERTILITY AND TRADITIONAL CHINESE MEDICINE: A Laywoman's Guide
by Bob Flaws
ISBN 0-936185-14-7

THE ESSENCE OF LIU FENG-WU'S GYNECOLOGY
by Liu Feng-wu,
translated by Yang Shou-zhong
ISBN 0-936185-88-0

EXTRA TREATISES BASED ON INVESTIGATION & INQUIRY: A Translation of Zhu Dan-xi's Ge Zhi Yu Lun
translation by Yang Shou-zhong
ISBN 0-936185-53-8

FIRE IN THE VALLEY: TCM Diagnosis & Treatment of Vaginal Diseases
by Bob Flaws
ISBN 0-936185-25-2

FU QING-ZHU'S GYNECOLOGY
trans. by Yang Shou-zhong and Liu Da-wei
ISBN 0-936185-35-X

FULFILLING THE ESSENCE: A Handbook of Traditional & Contemporary Treatments for Female Infertility
by Bob Flaws
ISBN 0-936185-48-1

GOLDEN NEEDLE WANG LE-TING: A 20th Century Master's Approach to Acupuncture
by Yu Hui-chan and Han Fu-ru, trans. by Shuai Xue-zhong

A GUIDE TO GYNECOLOGY
by Ye Heng-yin, trans. by Bob Flaws and Shuai Xue-zhong
ISBN 1-891845-19-5

A HANDBOOK OF TCM PATTERNS & TREATMENTS
by Bob Flaws & Daniel Finney
ISBN 0-936185-70-8

A HANDBOOK OF TRADITIONAL CHINESE DERMATOLOGY
by Liang Jian-hui, trans. by Zhang Ting-liang & Bob Flaws
ISBN 0-936185-07-4

A HANDBOOK OF TRADITIONAL CHINESE GYNECOLOGY
by Zhejiang College of TCM, trans. by Zhang Ting-liang & Bob Flaws
ISBN 0-936185-06-6 (4th edit.)

A HANDBOOK OF CHINESE HEMATOLOGY
by Simon Becker
ISBN 1-891845-16-0

A HANDBOOK OF MENSTRUAL DISEASES IN CHINESE MEDICINE
by Bob Flaws
ISBN 0-936185-82-1

A HANDBOOK of TCM PEDIATRICS
by Bob Flaws
ISBN 0-936185-72-4

A HANDBOOK OF TCM UROLOGY & MALE SEXUAL DYSFUNCTION
by Anna Lin, OMD
ISBN 0-936185-36-8

THE HEART & ESSENCE OF DAN-XI'S METHODS OF TREATMENT
by Xu Dan-xi, trans. by Yang Shou-zhong
ISBN 0-926185-49-X

THE HEART TRANSMISSION OF MEDICINE
by Liu Yi-ren, trans. by Yang Shou-zhong
ISBN 0-936185-83-X

HIGHLIGHTS OF ANCIENT ACUPUNCTURE PRESCRIPTIONS
trans. by Honora Lee Wolfe & Rose Crescenz
ISBN 0-936185-23-6

IMPERIAL SECRETS OF HEALTH & LONGEVITY
by Bob Flaws
ISBN 0-936185-51-1

INSIGHTS OF A SENIOR ACUPUNCTURIST
by Miriam Lee
ISBN 0-936185-33-3

KEEPING YOUR CHILD HEALTHY WITH CHINESE MEDICINE
by Bob Flaws
ISBN 0-936185-71-6

THE LAKESIDE MASTER'S STUDY OF THE PULSE
by Li Shi-zhen, trans. by Bob Flaws
ISBN 1-891845-01-2

MASTER TONG'S ACUPUNCTURE
by Miriam Lee
ISBN 0-926185-37-6

THE MEDICAL I CHING: Oracle of the Healer Within
by Miki Shima
ISBN 0-936185-38-4

MANAGING MENOPAUSE NATURALLY with Chinese Medicine
by Honora Lee Wolfe
ISBN 0-936185-98-8

PAO ZHI: Introduction to Processing Chinese Medicinals to Enhance Their Therapeutic Effect
by Philippe Sionneau
ISBN 0-936185-62-1

PATH OF PREGNANCY, VOL. I, Gestational Disorders
by Bob Flaws
ISBN 0-936185-39-2

PATH OF PREGNANCY, Vol. II, Postpartum Diseases
by Bob Flaws
ISBN 0-936185-42-2

THE PULSE CLASSIC: A Translation of the Mai Jing
by Wang Shu-he, trans. by Yang Shou-zhong
ISBN 0-936185-75-9

SEVENTY ESSENTIAL CHINESE HERBAL FORMULAS
by Bob Flaws
ISBN 0-936185-59-7

SHAOLIN SECRET FORMULAS for Treatment of External Injuries
by De Chan, trans. by Zhang Ting-liang & Bob Flaws
ISBN 0-936185-08-2

STATEMENTS OF FACT IN TRADITIONAL CHINESE MEDICINE
by Bob Flaws
ISBN 0-936185-52-X

STICKING TO THE POINT 1: A Rational Methodology for the Step by Step Formulation & Administration of an Acupuncture Treatment
by Bob Flaws
ISBN 0-936185-17-1

STICKING TO THE POINT 2: A Study of Acupuncture & Moxibustion Formulas and Strategies
by Bob Flaws
ISBN 0-936185-97-X

A STUDY OF DAOIST ACUPUNCTURE
by Liu Zheng-cai
ISBN 1-891845-08-X

TEACH YOURSELF TO READ MODERN MEDICAL CHINESE
by Bob Flaws
ISBN 0-936185-99-6

THE SYSTEMATIC CLASSIC OF ACUPUNCTURE & MOXIBUSTION A translation of the Jia Yi Jing
by Huang-fu Mi, trans. by Yang Shou-zhong & Charles Chace
ISBN 0-936185-29-5

THE TAO OF HEALTHY EATING ACCORDING TO CHINESE MEDICINE
by Bob Flaws
ISBN 0-936185-92-9

THE TREATMENT OF DISEASE IN TCM, Vol I: Diseases of the Head & Face Including Mental/Emotional Disorders
by Philippe Sionneau & Lü Gang
ISBN 0-936185-69-4

THE TREATMENT OF DISEASE IN TCM, Vol. II: Diseases of the Eyes, Ears, Nose, & Throat
by Sionneau & Lü
ISBN 0-936185-69-4

THE TREATMENT OF DISEASE, Vol. III: Diseases of the Mouth, Lips, Tongue, Teeth & Gums
by Sionneau & Lü
ISBN 0-936185-79-1

THE TREATMENT OF DISEASE, Vol IV: Diseases of the Neck, Shoulders, Back, & Limbs
by Philippe Sionneau & Lü Gang
ISBN 0-936185-89-9

THE TREATMENT OF DISEASE, Vol V: Diseases of the Chest & Abdomen
by Philippe Sionneau & Lü Gang
ISBN 1-891845-02-0

THE TREATMENT OF DISEASE, Vol VI: Diseases of the Urogential System & Proctology
by Philippe Sionneau & Lü Gang
ISBN 1-891845-05-5

THE TREATMENT OF DISEASE, Vol VII: General Symptoms
by Philippe Sionneau & Lü Gang
ISBN 1-891845-14-4

THE TREATMENT OF EXTERNAL DISEASES WITH ACUPUNCTURE & MOXIBUSTION
by Yan Cui-lan and Zhu Yun-long, trans. by Yang Shou-zhong
ISBN 0-936185-80-5

THE TREATMENT OF MODERN WESTERN MEDICAL DISEASES WITH CHINESE MEDICINE
by Bob Flaws & Philippe Sionneau
ISBN 1-891845-20-9

THE TREATMENT OF DIABETES MELLITUS WITH CHINESE MEDICINE
by Bob Flaws, Lynn Kuchinski & Robert Casañas, M.D.
ISBN 1-891845-21-7

160 ESSENTIAL CHINESE HERBAL PATENT MEDICINES
by Bob Flaws
ISBN 1-891945-12-8

630 QUESTIONS & ANSWERS ABOUT CHINESE HERBAL MEDICINE: A Workbook & Study Guide
by Bob Flaws
ISBN 1-891845-04-7

230 ESSENTIAL CHINESE MEDICINALS
by Bob Flaws
ISBN 1-891845-03-9